Foreword

The National Food Survey is the longest running continuous survey of household food consumption in the world. Over a period of 50 years, the Survey has provided a wide range of information which has contributed to the analysis of policy and to monitoring the change in the diets of British households.

This volume represents the edited proceedings of a symposium to mark 'Fifty Years of the National Food Survey'. The proceedings not only provide an insight into the origins of the Survey but also into how the national diet has changed. They also show how the Survey has adapted to capture these changes accurately while retaining continuity in the data which is a unique feature of the National Food Survey.

As the current chairman of the National Food Survey Committee which advises on the running of the Survey, I would like to pay tribute to the dedication and foresight of all those who have contributed to the Survey over its lifespan. Many committee members spanning this period participated in the Symposium; special thanks are due to Miss Dorothy Hollingsworth and Dr Arnold Baines, who were associated with the Survey in its early years, and to the Food Minister, David Maclean, who gave the opening address at the Symposium.

Finally, I would like to say that the National Food Survey is continuing to move forward and to adapt to changing conditions. Details are given within this volume of important developments designed to keep the Survey up to date. In particular, plans are in hand to obtain information on the increasing proportion of food purchased and consumed away from the home.

R.E.MORDUE

Chairman, National Food Survey Committee

Biographical Notes

DAVID MACLEAN, MP
Parliamentary Secretary in MAFF, with special responsibility for food

DR ARNOLD BAINES
Formerly Chief Statistician in MAFF, Joint Secretary to the National Food Survey (NFS) Committee 1954-1961, Member of the NFS Committee 1961-1985

MISS DOROTHY HOLLINGSWORTH
Joint Secretary to the NFS Committee from its inception until 1966, member of the NFS Committee 1966-1985. Second Director General of the British Nutrition Foundation

PROFESSOR CHRISTOPHER RITSON
Professor of Agricultural Marketing, University of Newcastle-upon-Tyne

RICHARD HUTCHINS
Postgraduate student, University of Newcastle-upon-Tyne

DR DAVID BUSS
Head of MAFF's Nutrition Branch, Joint Secretary to the NFS Committee

PROFESSOR ANDREW CHESHER
Professor of Econometrics, University of Bristol

DR JOHN SLATER
Senior Economic Advisor and Head of Economics and Statistics (Food) Division, MAFF with overall responsibility for the NFS

DR MARTIN WISEMAN
Senior Medical Officer, Department of Health

ROBERT W WENLOCK
Principal Research Officer, Department of Health

IVOR HUNT
Director of Marketing Services, J Sainsbury plc

DR LESLEY YEOMANS
Director of External Affairs, Tate and Lyle Speciality Sweeteners. Previously with the Consumers' Association

ROBERT REDPATH
Principal Social Survey Officer, Social Survey Division, Office of Population Censuses and Surveys

MAFF

**Ministry of Agriculture
Fisheries and Food**

Fifty Years
of the
National Food Survey
1940 - 1990

The proceedings of a symposium
held in December 1990, London

Edited by Dr J M Slater

LONDON : HMSO

© Crown Copyright 1991
Applications for reproduction should
be made to HMSO
First published 1991

ISBN 0 11 242909 2

Printed in the United Kingdom for HMSO
Dd293410 7/91 C12 G3390 10170

Acknowledgements

Many contributed to the success of the Symposium and to the production of this edited version of the proceedings. Thanks are due first to those who provided papers drawing on their particular expertise and knowledge of the Survey. The organisational arrangements owed much to the efforts of the staff of the National Food Survey branch. In particular, Sheila Dixon, Carolyn Hamilton, Melanie Smith and my secretary, Linda West, worked unstintingly on the detailed arrangements and on setting up the proceedings for printing.

EDITOR

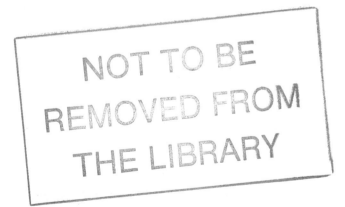

Table of Contents

List of Tables and Figures

page

SECTION IV The Value of the National Food Survey

SECTION V Planned Changes to the National Food Survey

Food Policy
and the
National Food Survey

CHAPTER 1

Food Policy and the National Food Survey

David Maclean

Introduction

I am delighted to be contributing to this Symposium to mark the 50th Anniversary of the National Food Survey. There are many landmarks relating to *agricultural* statistics and, indeed, one of our contributors - Dr Arnold Baines - is the author of a *A Century of Agricultural Statistics* [1]. It is, however, fitting that this landmark in the history of *food* statistics falls at a time when such great emphasis is being placed on food policy.

I have found it fascinating to look back at the work that went on in MAFF 50 years ago. The publications from that time illustrate just how ingenious those responsible for our food policy were at a time of acute food shortages and without the benefit of the technology we have today. Indeed, a second contribution is from Dorothy Hollingsworth who, as a nutritionist, was responsible for advising on dietary requirements and was closely associated with the National Food Survey (NFS) for many years. Then, as now, the NFS played an important role in measuring and monitoring the changes in the diet of households in Great Britain.

Comparison with the 1940s

Policy is, of course, a continuous process. It means evaluating scientific research and appraising other advice. It also means setting specific objectives and formulating programmes to meet them. After that, we have to monitor the outcome. In the 1940s, scientific research was mainly directed to agricultural production. Food policy objectives were limited to making sure we had an adequate minimum diet given the supply of food available. Until the NFS was set up, monitoring even these objectives was extremely limited.

Many of the basic foods that were bought in 1940 are similar to those recorded in the Survey today. But the pattern of consumption has radically changed. We eat less carcase meat, less sugar and less bread but more fruit and vegetables (Table 1.1).

Table 1.1
Household consumption
of principal foods

ounces per person per week

	1941-1946	1965-1969	1985-1989
Carcase meat	14.00	16.55	12.73
Fish	7.18	5.70	5.08
Bread	60.50	39.06	30.42
Milk (pints)	4.10	5.22	4.03
Butter	2.08	6.13	2.20
Eggs (no.)	2.18	4.71	2.80
Fruit	12.48	30.08	30.64
Potatoes	67.78	52.15	37.88
Other vegetables	35.96	34.17	46.13
Sugar	8.78	16.87	7.47

However, I want to single out what I see as two of the most significant factors about household food purchases today compared with those of 1940. The first is the much greater range of food items, produced to very high standards, available to households today. In a modern supermarket, consumers can choose from well over 5,000 different food items.

One cannot but be impressed, for instance, by the range and quality of the fruit and vegetables available to us today. And the increased purchases of fruit and vegetables have contributed to a healthier diet. Few consumers would wish to return to the diet of the 1940s which was described in the second report of the National Food Survey Committee [2] as 'somewhat dull' - something of an understatement.

The second significant fact is that, whereas 50 years ago households had to spend about a third of their income on buying the food they needed, the proportion today is less than 12 per cent (Figure 1.2).

Figure 1.2
Household expenditure
on food as a percentage
of total consumers'
expenditure

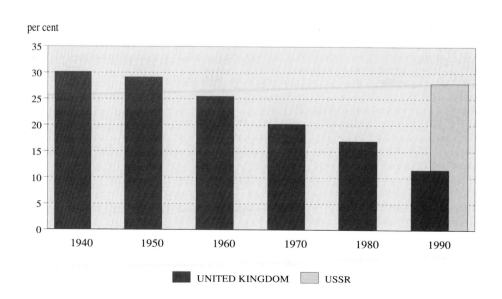

4

This leaves consumers with significantly more of their income to spend on other goods and services. This position in the United Kingdom(UK) today is, of course, a far cry from that in the planned economies. The average consumer in the USSR has been in much the same position in 1990 as the British consumer was 50 years ago.

Formulation of food policy

These two factors reflect the significant achievements of food policies over the last 50 years and, in particular, in the last 10 years. But policy is a continuous process and I want to turn now to the Government's food policies. They are policies built on scientific research, on expert advice and on listening to, and learning from, consumers. It reflects the Government's emphasis on achieving an adequate supply of safe and nutritious food at reasonable prices. These policies are, I believe, more comprehensive than ever before during peacetime. And yet they provide flexibility to meet changing needs.

Research

For example, let us look at how the Government support for food research is being re-focused towards work on food safety and nutrition. In 1991-1992, MAFF will be spending a further £3.7 million over and above the £11 million which the department is already spending on research in food safety and applied nutrition.

Of course this is only a small fraction of overall Government expenditure in these areas. There is also substantial investment by the Research Councils and by other departments, notably the Department of Health. Together with MAFF's expenditure, this amounts to some £35 million; and the food industry has also increased its research enormously.

Expenditure on food safety research represents an investment which will put the UK at the forefront of protecting the interests of the consumer. Much of the new resource which Government is making available will be in the area of nutrition. In this area MAFF has, in conjunction with the Department of Health, sought to lay down the following priorities:

- Cardiovascular disease;

- Cancer;

- Osteoporosis;

- Nutritional standards for the elderly;

- Optimal nutrition;

- Surveillance methodology.

This reflects the determination of Government departments to work together to target the research on important public health issues relating to the national diet. In particular, we will be looking to support major new research initiatives on the role of dietary fat in atherogenesis and heart disease; on dietary calcium intake in adolescents and its relation to bone strength and on the levels and type of fibre intake which are consistent with meeting health and nutrition goals.

None of this research can be effectively implemented unless we understand the factors that influence consumers' choice of food and the changing nature of consumer habits. Work will be commissioned in this area to understand how best to implement nutrition policy. We want our consumers to be given sound advice on healthy eating - advice based on scientific research and analysis - not on assertions or minority self-interests.

There is a similar programme of research in the area of food microbiology and there are comprehensive programmes of research on pesticides and other residues and on controlling animal diseases, such as brucellosis, BSE and salmonella. Particular examples include the work on developing rapid diagnostic tests for salmonella enteritidis infection in poultry; tests for BSE based on the detection of prior protein deposits - some £4.9 million has been earmarked for research on BSE in 1991-92 - and studying the survival and growth of pathogenic bacteria. In fact, wherever there is seen to be a problem or potential problem on food safety, steps are taken to ensure that any necessary research is undertaken.

Of course research, both in the UK and elsewhere, must be properly evaluated and targeted. Ministers are advised by many scientific and technical committees to ensure that this happens. The diagram illustrates the range of advice available (Figure 1.3).

Figure 1.3
Structure of main
advisory committees

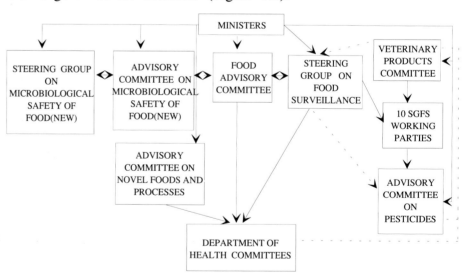

Solid lines between committees indicate formal links and broken lines show informal connections

As with the NFS, membership of expert committees is designed to provide balanced advice from experts and from lay persons. This is illustrated by the membership of the Food Advisory Committee which comprises:

Chairman   Vice-Chancellor
14 members   5 from Industry
                4 from Research / Medical Institutions
                3 from Consumers
                2 Food Law Enforcement Experts

Of course, there are other special committees. And I must mention a committee under the chairmanship of Sir Mark Richmond which has been looking at the microbiological safety of food [3]. Our decision to establish this committee early is a good example of the Government's commitment to tackling particular problems as they arise. The recommendations which the committee made early this year have been published and are being implemented. Our response includes establishing permanent advisory and surveillance arrangements, and more will be said about these later.

Policy co-ordination

To ensure that all relevant advice and all policy recommendations are co-ordinated and implemented effectively, the Minister of Agriculture set up, in 1989, the Food Safety Directorate (Figure 1.4).

Figure 1.4
Food Safety Directorate

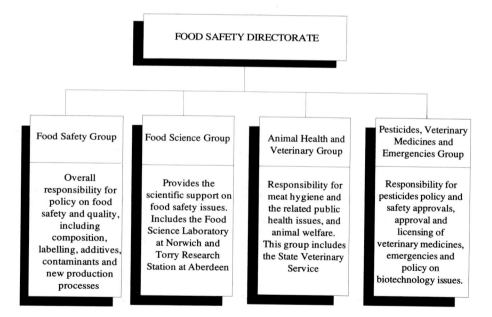

This new directorate brings together, under the overall control of the Food Minister, all food safety work for which the Ministry is responsible. It has allowed the Ministry not only to channel its resources more effectively into maintaining the safety and quality of the nation's food supplies but also to provide an important forum for consulting consumers. A key event in this consultation was the establishment, also in 1989, of a new Consumers Panel. The Panel, which the Food Minister chairs, is made up of ordinary consumers nominated by the main consumer bodies but appointed in an individual capacity. The Panel's terms of reference are to review matters relating to the implementation of food safety policies and to examine issues of concern to consumers. The Panel has already achieved a very useful exchange of views and ideas, and I look forward to even greater achievements in the future.

The Food Safety Act   A further indication of the commitment to a co-ordinated food policy has been in the close working links MAFF has with the Department of Health. This is invaluable when questions of food safety legislation have to be addressed as witnessed with the work in respect of the Food Safety Act [4]. This Act represents a major re-think of our national food laws. At the same time, the opportunity was taken to make sure that the Government had the right powers to operate within the European Community (EC) legal framework, which will be increasingly important to manufacturers and traders in the run up to 1992. The Single Market will be a challenge extending right across industry and it will also have significant implications for enforcement authorities as the EC moves towards consumer standards.

The new Act has been designed to give a highly flexible framework, allowing detailed controls to be put in place as they become needed. In that way, regulations can keep pace with technological developments, for example, either in the way foods are prepared or in the way they are distributed and stored. That flexibility also allows regulations to be made covering the whole food chain from farm to shop or restaurant table. Some of the basic laws have been changed to give better consumer protection, and there are improved provisions concerning food safety enforcement to make it more effective than ever before.

The Food Safety Act, and initial regulations needed to make it fully workable in practice, come into effect on 1 January 1991. These regulations will cover some technical matters such as qualifications for public analysts and food examiners, division of enforcement responsibilities, and rules on sampling for analysis or examination, as well as measures for control of food irradiation facilities and rules for labelling irradiated food.

The Department of Health will be consulting shortly on proposals for regulations setting requirements for training those who handle food. That Department will also circulate proposals for the registration by local authorities of premises used commercially for the preparation of food.

The Act contains powers for Ministers to issue Codes of Practice for food authorities, and the first of these will come into operation on 1 January 1991. The Codes will help ensure that enforcement standards can be made evenly across the country, and if necessary Ministers will be able to direct authorities to comply. The Codes have been developed with the help of an Implementation Advisory Committee made up of experts from both central and local government with experience of enforcement matters.

In summary, the objective of the Act is to provide a balanced package of measures that can safeguard the consumer with the minimum burdens on industry. The Government is providing extra resources to help the enforcement authorities discharge the new responsibilities placed on them by the legislation. There is an underlying commitment that the safety of consumers must come above any other consideration.

Keeping the food industry and consumers informed

The structure now in place enables policies to be reviewed by Ministers who need to take the right decisions to promote the highest standards of food safety. It also provides flexibility to introduce policy changes in the light of new evidence. However, the underlying principles will not change. The first of these is to ensure that food is safe. The second is to ensure that the consumer has the information needed to choose a healthy and nutritious diet.

Policies cannot be effective unless the industry and the consumer are properly informed. MAFF undertakes a wide range of campaigns for this purpose and over half the department's publicity budget is deployed to this end. Campaigns are targeted at those who supply the consumer - the food manufacturers, the food retailers and the catering trade - and also at the consumer, from school children to those who do the shopping and prepare the meals.

In particular, advice is given on action which needs to be taken to ensure that food is safe and also to explain Government safeguards in respect of additives, pesticides and animal medicines. These campaigns make use of books, videos, exhibitions and advertising as necessary. Some broadly based campaigns like the 'Food Sense' series are aimed at the public and the food industry and use all these media.

Particular emphasis is put on the second underlying principle of ensuring that consumers have sufficient information so that they can choose, from the wide range of foods available, a diet which suits them. The department liaises closely with the Department of Health and the Health Education Authority on all matters of diet and health. A recent joint publication 'Eight Guidelines for a Healthy Diet' [5] provides clear, sound, overall dietary advice which can be related to people's everyday lives, and campaigns such as the HEA led 'Look After Your Heart' programme, are aimed at further encouraging healthier diets.

Food labelling

Linked in with this are the steps we take to ensure that food is clearly and informatively labelled. We were one of the first countries within the EC to introduce a system for nutrition labelling of foods and have played a leading role in negotiating the EC's Nutrition Labelling (Rules) Directive [6] which builds on the UK's 1987 guidelines and which enables consumers to make an informed choice about the food they buy. The new EC Directive lays down a statutory nutritional labelling format. In general the provisions are voluntary unless particular claims are made. Already very many foods carry nutrition declarations and we are continuing to encourage manufacturers and retailers to provide as much information as possible in accordance with the provisions of the Directive, even though it does not have to be implemented for some time yet. This is an example of an area where the Government is giving every encouragement to manufacturers and retailers to take a positive approach to letting consumers have the information well in advance of the legislation. Advice and education presented in the clearest possible terms that avoid confusion are every bit as important as statutory controls.

Labelling is one of the most effective ways of informing and educating the public. A recent consumer survey was commissioned to establish just what it is that consumers look for on a label, and whether what they get is clear and easy to understand. The Food Advisory Committee (FAC) is now considering the survey results as part of its thorough review of food labelling law and the FAC report is expected very shortly [7].

Let the consumer decide

(a) **Nutrition monitoring:** To fulfil its responsibilities, government does need to know what people are eating, what it costs, and the amounts of nutrients and other constituents in their foods and diets. For 50 years now, the NFS has played a very important part in our surveillance programme. It was originally set up to monitor the effectiveness of the Government's wartime food policies; it then monitored the changes at the end of rationing, the changes that arose as people chose to buy more pre-packed foods, the effects of the inflation in the 1970s, and now the effects of the comparatively recent interest in diet and health. Have people changed their diets? If so, has everybody changed, and in what ways? Have the changes improved the nutritional quality of the diet or not?

MAFF undertakes many detailed studies of special groups of people to check very specific points. These include the following:

- National Food Survey;

- Dietary habits of 15 to 25 year olds [8];

- Dietary and nutritional survey of British adults [9];

- Dietary survey of infants 6 to 12 months
  (Not yet published);

- Dietary survey of pre-school children
  (To be undertaken in 1991-1992).

Recently a new programme was started to monitor all the foods that individuals eat and, with the Department of Health, to check their health too. But these surveys are very time consuming and expensive and it is difficult to ensure that the results are fully representative. By contrast, the NFS is not only truly national, but it also accurately measures all the food coming into the home. And the results are available quickly! Quarterly results are available about six weeks after the end of the survey period and full year results are published in the annual reports of the NFS Committee [10].

The nutritional results have always been of central importance. We have long been able to check whether the recommended amounts of minerals and vitamins were being met. Gradually the range of nutrients covered has been extended in response to new interests and concerns. For instance, the main types of fatty acids are covered, not just the total amount of fat. Sodium, fibre and sugars have also been added to the nutrients measured and further minerals and vitamins will be added soon.

The Department of Health, as well as MAFF, have made use of these results in many significant reports on public health. They were used in COMA's reports [11,12] on the relationships between diet and cardiovascular disease. NFS results have also been used to determine the contribution that fortified foods make to people's nutrient intakes and to see the value of maintaining our present food fortification policies for flour and margarine. Most recently the results have been used to help set scientifically sound Dietary Reference Values (DRVs) of nutrients for the United Kingdom. This latter report is due to be published in 1991.

Of course the NFS is not only used for monitoring nutritional trends. The Survey has a significant role in monitoring economic trends. Data from the Survey are used in the construction of national accounts and for other economic indicators, including the Retail Price Index. The results supplement other measures of the need for, and availability of, food supplies, and provide information on which the impact of economic policies can be monitored and evaluated. In other words, the NFS contributes to the objective of ensuring adequate supplies of food at reasonable prices as well as to the monitoring of nutritional trends.

(b) Chemical surveillance: While the NFS has a central role in our programme of monitoring and surveillance, the department also has an extensive and vitally important programme in respect of food safety. Surveillance of the chemical safety of the food supply is a key part of our scientific work to protect the consumer. For many years Government scientists have carried out work to quantify the amounts of nutrients, additives and chemical contaminants in our diet. This high quality scientific work covers a wide range of substances - from aflatoxins to veterinary residues. Its purpose is to identify problems and to ensure that they are solved.

Food chemical surveillance is co-ordinated by the Steering Group on Food Surveillance, an internationally respected group whose work is acknowledged as the best in Europe. Detailed work is carried out by ten working parties reporting to the Steering Group, each of which covers a particular area in the range of topics falling under the Steering Group's remit. This key scientific work is reported to the public in a series of reports - Food Surveillance papers [13]. These reports have covered important topics such as future work on food composition and intake. All of the work carried out by the Steering Group is made publicly available.

This important work helps Government ensure that there is a constant supply of safe food to keep the consumer properly fed and nourished. The key to much of the work is to look for problems before they occur and then to check that any necessary action has the desired effect. It is through this pro-active approach that food surveillance contributes to the science of food safety.

(c) Microbiological food surveillance: To complement the work carried out in the field of food chemical surveillance, it was announced earlier this year that a national microbiological food surveillance and assessment system is to be established. This will be based on a new independent Advisory Committee and a new Steering Group on the Microbiological Safety of Food and gives effect to the recommendations of the Committee on the Microbiological Safety of Food, chaired by Sir Mark Richmond [3].

The Steering Group will manage surveillance and research and will present policy conclusions to Ministers. It will consist both of officials and of experts from outside Government.

The Advisory Committee will bring outside expertise to bear on the interpretation of the results of surveillance and on the policy formation process. This Committee will have an entirely independent membership and chairman, who will be chosen for their expertise and invited from relevant backgrounds including consumer interests.

The establishment of this national microbiologial surveillance and assessment system will ensure a more co-ordinated, effective and responsive long-term policy on microbiological food safety. I hope that this in turn will lead to increased public confidence in the safety of food.

A comprehensive food strategy

Some have criticised Britain for not having an all embracing food and nutrition policy with narrowly defined objectives. I think you will agree that this criticism is misplaced.

- We have policies to help ensure that the farming industry and the food industry provide an abundant, safe and nutritious food supply.

- These policies are designed to ensure that all sectors of the population have access to the food they want at reasonable cost.

- And that the special nutritional needs of vulnerable groups are identified and met.

- We have an active research programme not only on food supplies and food safety but on the relationships between diet and disease.

- Expert advice is available and account is taken of new evidence.

- There are educational programmes to disseminate advice and to encourage the population to choose healthy diets. This advice has to recognise the different physiological and cultural needs of groups such as the young, the elderly and the ethnic communities.

- Food labelling policies are designed to help consumers to understand the nutritional value of the foods they eat. And to prevent misleading claims.

- Finally we have comprehensive surveillance programmes to monitor the effectiveness of policies.

Today, British consumers have a wider choice of safe and nutritious foods than ever before. They also live longer and are in better health. This is being achieved by having a comprehensive, but flexible, set of policies which allow us to meet new situations on food safety and nutrition as they arise.

Changes to the National Food Survey

I have pointed out the need for expert advice, the need for flexibility and the need to keep up to date. The NFS embraces all of these. The NFS has established itself over a period of 50 years as one of the most authoritative household food surveys in the world. It owes this authority to the care and dedication of successive members of the NFS Committee and their efforts to ensure the continuing relevance of the data collected and the statistical reliability of the results.

However, Ministers have also recognised the need to keep the Survey up to date. Dr Yeomans will draw attention to a recent review of certain aspects of the NFS and changes that are planned. These changes will be aimed not only at ensuring that the results remain statistically valid but also that account is taken of the changing food scene, especially in respect of the increasing amount of food consumed away from the home.

It is a daunting task to look forward to food policy in the next 50 years. However, we will not go far wrong if we can count on the sort of continuity, combined with adaptation to change, that has been provided by the National Food Survey over the last 50 years.

REFERENCES

[1] Ministry of Agriculture, Fisheries and Food (1968), *A Century of Agricultural Statistics, GB, 1866-1966*, HMSO.

[2] Ministry of Agriculture, Fisheries and Food (1951), *Studies in Urban Household Diets 1944-49*, second report of the National Food Survey Committee, HMSO.

[3] Richmond, Sir Mark (1990), *The Microbiological Safety of Food, Part I*, report of the Committee on the Microbiological Safety of Food, HMSO.

[4] HMSO (1990) *Food Safety Act.*

[5] Department of Health (1990) *Eight Guidelines for a Healthy Diet*, Food Sense Series, HMSO.

[6] Official Journal of the European Communities (1990), *Nutrition Labelling (Rules) Directive, 90/496/EEC*, 6 October, 276/40, Luxembourg.

[7] Food Advisory Committee (1989), *Nutritional Claims in Food Labelling and Advertising*, HMSO.

[8] Bull, N.L. (1985),*Dietary Habits of 15 to 25-Year-Olds*, Human Nutrition; Applied Nutrition, Vol 39A, Supplement 1.

[9] Gregory, J. et al. (1990) *The Dietary and Nutritional Survey of British Adults*, Office of Population Censuses and Surveys, HMSO.

[10] Ministry of Agriculture, Fisheries and Food (1990), *Household Food Consumption and Expenditure, 1989*, annual report of the National Food Survey Committee, HMSO.

[11] Department of Health and Social Security (1974) *Diet and Coronary Heart Disease*, HMSO.

[12] Department of Health and Social Security (1984), *Diet and Cardiovascular Disease*, HMSO.

[13] Ministry of Agriculture, Fisheries and Food (1978-90), *Food Surveillance Papers, 1-30*, HMSO.

Historical Perspectives of the National Food Survey

CHAPTER 2

How the National Food Survey Began

Arnold Baines

Introduction

This year we can celebrate two distinct anniversaries. In January 1950, the National Food Survey (NFS) of Great Britain achieved the national coverage which its name connotes. It has provided the Ministry and the public with quarterly estimates of household food consumption and expenditure for the past forty years; but it was the immediate successor of the Wartime Food Survey (from 1945 the Family Food Survey) of urban working-class households, which began in July 1940, so that this year is also and primarily a fiftieth anniversary, a golden jubilee. But we must start a few years further back, since that Survey, like the Ministry of Food itself, had three progenitors.

The first was the Market Supply Committee, set up in 1934 by the Agricultural Departments to bring together information on the food position of Britain, especially on total requirements in relation to market supply and the effect on consumption of changes in price. Perhaps it was the reference to requirements which stimulated the Health Departments, and our second antecessor was the Advisory Committee on Nutrition, set up by the Health Ministers in 1935 to inquire into the diet of the people and to report on changes therein which appeared desirable on nutritional grounds. They drew upon the data available to the Market Supply Committee, and their first report in 1937 [1] made some far-reaching suggestions, notably that the consumption of liquid milk should be doubled and consumption of fruit and vegetables increased. Their scale of nutritional requirements was that suggested by the Technical Committee of the League of Nations Health Organisation.

Meanwhile, in 1936 a Food (Defence Plans) Department had been created within the Board of Trade to formulate plans for the supply, control and distribution of food in an emergency. Its report in 1938 [2] was the basis of the organisation and policy of the Ministry of Food, which was set up as soon as war was declared on Hitler's Germany. There had been a common underlying assumption from 1936 onwards that a wartime government would have to assume responsibility for supplies and prices at least to the extent reached in 1918.

Accordingly, during the 'phoney war' period from September 1939 to May 1940, stocks were requisitioned and the Ministry of Food became the sole importer of the main foodstuffs and sole buyer from the farmer. Registration for rationing began in November, and actual rationing in January, together with food subsidies to offset what would otherwise have been the effect on consumer prices of the heavy losses which the Ministry was sustaining.

The pace of administrative change accelerated with the collapse of France. Cheap or free milk was provided for young children and expectant mothers, and the school meals service was rapidly expanded. Canteen meals were encouraged and then required. British Restaurants were established during the Battle of Britain. By early 1941, there was effectively full employment, with large increases in wages, so that demand grew while supplies from overseas dwindled. There was an intensified drive to secure the expansion of home-produced food, especially potatoes and cereals. The Government undertook to subsidise the principal articles of consumption so as to hold the Cost of Living Index within the range of 25 to 30 per cent above the level of 1 September 1939. The pattern of rationing, price control and food supplies was set, and most remarkably it was maintained for the rest of the war, thanks to the Lend-Lease agreement with the United States, the start of the special economic relationship. By the end of 1941, it was the consensus of Ministers and the public that the immediate food crisis had been surmounted, or rather that it had been knowingly deferred until the war ended.

Precursors of the NFS

From the outbreak of war, and indeed before that, it was generally accepted in Whitehall that the Government would need to know what was actually happening to consumers, which might not be what legislators and administrators prescribed or intended. In the words of a former Minister of Agriculture, the choice was between discussions taken in ignorance and those based on knowledge. The Health and Agricultural Departments and the incipient Ministry of Food were well aware of the intrinsic importance of the various budgetary and consumption enquiries which had been undertaken during the 1930s, and of their impact on public opinion. Four of these were regarded as representing the urban working-class households on which attention was concentrated. The first was Boyd Orr's *Food, Health and Income* [3] begun in 1932 in the depression, when real incomes were at their lowest; its budgets were collected in spring and early summer, and were overweighted by the industrial north and by large families.

Crawford and Broadley's *The People's Food* [4] was more representative; it covered seven large towns between October 1936 and March 1937. During 1937-38, the Ministry of Labour, in the course of rebasing the Cost of Living Index, placed a log-book to record a week's food expenditure with 21,000 households in October, and asked the same households to repeat the exercise in January, April and July. Eventually some 9,000 family budgets covering the four seasons were secured. Finally, the Rowett Research Institute carried out a more precise dietary enquiry, called the Carnegie Survey from its sponsor, between January 1937 and April 1939, taking account of stock changes and making allowance for wastage. This survey provided a record of quantities suitable for comparison with the later wartime results in terms of nutrients [5].

The Wartime Food Survey

All these enquiries influenced the planning and design of the Wartime Food Survey, which was launched in July 1940, just after the fall of France, the time of our greatest peril and our greatest national unity. The object of the Survey was to assist the Government to decide on measures needed to anticipate food shortages and to mitigate their effect. The Survey was not intended at the time to provide a continuous record of national food consumption. Households in working class wards in seven cities were asked to record quantities of food purchased, or obtained from gardens or allotments or as gifts, during seven full days. The field workers also secured particulars of meals eaten away from home, or served to visitors, and ascertained the sex, age and occupation of all persons in the household. A 'household' comprised those persons for whom the informant (the 'housewife') catered, and a 'person' was defined as one who had at least 16 meals in the house during the week. Questions about income were not included; an attempt to obtain particulars of income was later made on a sub-sample in 1943, but was soon abandoned. Particulars of sweets, chocolate, ice-cream and alcoholic and most soft drinks were not sought, as they would often not be known to the housewife.

Until 1942, the Survey did not record changes in larder stocks. It was and is a general finding that when households are under observation average quantities consumed exceed average quantities entering the household, to an extent varying with the food and with the season. This was attributed to the housewife's pattern of behaviour being perturbed by the time and trouble involved in keeping the log-book, but in any case a survey can hardly avoid drawing her or his attention to the availability of stocks. As Heisenberg would say, one cannot observe the situation without disturbing it.

The Survey began in seven large towns: London, Reading, Birmingham, Cardiff, Liverpool, Sheffield and Glasgow. Four more were added in 1941, but Liverpool had to be replaced by Warrington owing to heavy air-raids. Comparability over time was further affected by evacuation of children to the countryside, and by their return. The number of towns reached 22 in 1943, 25 in 1944 and 42 in 1945. It had been intended to obtain records from the same households quarter by quarter, but this was soon abandoned since the repeat samples contained an undue proportion of pensioners' households and of families with young children with the housewife at home. When she went out to work, she was often too busy to participate further.

Special samples

Before 1950, the only occasion when the Survey focused attention on households at a low economic level was in 1944, when a so-called 'special sample' of poorly accommodated households within the general sample was analysed. The defining conditions were back-to-back housing, no running water, no separate lavatory, overcrowding (more than two persons per room), alleyway access and bad repair. Any one such condition qualified. Before the war the corresponding underclass had been shown to exhibit large differences from the working class generally. By 1944, with all allowances for difficulties of comparison, there had been a great improvement in the diets of these poor households, absolutely and relatively, but some characteristic features were still present; a propensity for easily prepared meals, especially fried fish and chips, presumably because of lack of cooking facilities or skill; low consumption of green vegetables and especially of fruit. Purely economic factors and lack of facilities do not suffice to explain this. We must look to pre-war habits, when fruit in particular was regarded by many poorer households as an unattainable luxury. Such habits may go far back and are very slow to change. The old Cost of Living Index, which was being stabilised as a matter of policy, took no account of fruit. It was not included until the new Index of Retail Prices was eventually introduced in 1947.

In the years 1944 to 1946 and nine months of 1947, a separate sample of urban middle-class households was obtained; the term is inexact, the basis of the selection being location in middle-class wards of the towns surveyed, just as the main sample was taken from working-class wards, though households whose station in life was inappropriate to their location were distinguished and transferred. In the 1940s, middle-class characteristics included a garage, a maid, a gardener and even a telephone; being in a profession, or in management, or having earned at least £6 a week before the war. The results for these middle-class households were not published until 1956. The Secretaries of the NFS Committee at that time must accept some responsibility both for the delay and for the final publication, but we would submit that the exercise was well worthwhile. The remarkable narrowing of the class difference was partly due to narrowing of the price range, so that the levelling was more pronounced for expenditure than for consumption; but even for consumption there had been some decline for the middle-class, contrasted with the general improvement in the working-class diet. For both classes, the diet in 1944 was wholesome, adequate and rather dull.

The post-war years

The end of the war, and the somewhat prompt termination of Lend-Lease in August 1945, precipitated the expected food crisis. The peoples of the liberated and occupied countries had to be fed. Agriculture everywhere was suffering from acute shortages of labour, machinery and

20

fertilisers, and from generally adverse weather. Further, Britain was not the only country where standards of consumption well above pre-war levels were being clamorously demanded. These difficulties did not affect the tried and trusted Survey methods, but from October 1947 to March 1948 the normal Survey was interrupted; this was the only lengthy break in its continuity during the fifty years which we are commemorating. Even bread and potatoes had to be rationed, and, for what were justifiably claimed as policy reasons, fieldwork was concentrated on the households of heavy manual workers in five industries where heavy work was still general; agriculture, mining, building, metals (iron and steel and non-ferrous) and shipbuilding. It was feared that in these groups food shortages might be such as to reduce output. Local mines or factories supplied suitable addresses, and the samples were then extended by snowballing, households of the required type providing additional contacts. In January, the general sample was resumed for a month to provide a benchmark.

Heavy manual workers tend to have large families, and households with several earners were over-represented because of the non-random method of selection. Nevertheless, the results were found useful and moderately reassuring, though it was judged impracticable, then and later, to make a formal assessment of nutritional adequacy. The results have permanent value, coming from a time before mechanisation and automation had greatly diminished the importance of heavy manual labour, though even at that time energy expenditure must have varied widely within each of the industries.

Some of the occupational differences found were regional; for example, the shipbuilders were concentrated in Scotland and the North, metal working was associated with the Midlands, while the building workers' diets were broadly Southern. The farm workers' households departed most widely from the other groups and from the urban working-class norm; as was to be expected, they had high consumption of milk, cheese and bacon, but not of any other meat, or of fish. For all the groups, the energy and nutritive values were well above those for the general sample for January, which had been taken for comparison, though this did not hold for fat and the fat-soluble vitamins. The additional calories which these groups needed and obtained came from carbohydrate rather than fat.

An important source of information auxiliary to the Food Survey in the difficult post-war years was provided by changes in body weight, for the interpretation of which I defer to Dorothy Hollingsworth; but there is no doubt that between 1945 and 1947 there was some loss of weight in adults and retardation of growth in children.

Signs of improvement, and with it a gradual reversion to pre-war differences in consumption patterns, became apparent during 1948 not least because of Marshall Aid. In that year, the NFS Committee was set up to consider the available material and to make recommendations regarding its publication. The tenth and last year of the urban working-class surveys was to be 1949. For that year, there were to be thorough analyses by household composition and by region, and the regional results were further analysed for certain selected types of family to obtain what was regarded as a purer measure of strictly geographical differences. For households with a single earner the data were also tabulated by his or her occupation, classified as heavy manual, light manual or non-manual. Attention was then further concentrated on the couples with no children, those with two children in addition, and those with four or more children. It was found that different occupational groups of the same family composition showed differences which, though not insignificant, were dominated by the differences associated with family size. For this reason, this particular form of classification was not perpetuated when the Survey became national in January 1950.

The so-called second report of the NFS Committee [6], which was not published until 1956, incorporated all the special studies relating to the first decade of the Survey, but over half that Report related to the exhaustive analyses for the single year 1949. Regrettably, the physical difficulties of handling old and worn punched cards precluded any further analyses for the years from 1940 to 1943, which included the period of transition to rationing and government control of food supplies.

The decision to make the Survey truly national was reached because unless a complete cross-section of the population is taken the full impact of changes in supplies and prices cannot be assessed, either on the general population or on the different groups within it. The NFS annual report for 1950 [7], and its successors, included analyses of food consumption and expenditure, energy value and nutrient composition by social class and household composition. It was no longer assumed, as in the earlier war years, that the effectiveness of policy decisions or non-decisions would be sufficiently reflected in urban working-class households. The change was certainly not made too early. A general policy of easing and then removing controls was well under way during 1949, although by midsummer 1950 the Korean war brought relaxation of controls to a temporary halt.

Henceforth, social class was defined in terms of ranges of the gross income of the head of the household, as stated by the housewife or inferred from details of occupation. (The 'head' and the 'housewife' can of course be of either gender). The term 'social class' was deliberately adopted, as the emphasis was on social rather than strictly economic standing. The concept goes back through Crawford and Broadley to the usual practice of field investigations into marketing in the early 1930s.

Throughout its history, the National Food Survey has been extensively used in the daily work of the Ministry and the Government; but, without prejudice to this primary purpose, the availability of its findings has come to serve much wider interests. This Symposium is intended to illustrate its various uses, and perhaps to promote them.

REFERENCES

[1] Ministry of Health (1937), *First Report of the Advisory Committee on Nutrition*, HMSO.

[2] Board of Trade (1938), *Report of the Food (Defence Plans) Department for the year ended 31 December 1937*, HMSO.

[3] Orr, J B (1936), *Food, Health and Income*, MacMillan.

[4] Crawford, W E and Broadley, H (1938), *The People's Food*, Heinemann.

[5] Rowett Research Institute (1955), *Family Health and Diet in Pre-War Britain*, Carnegie UK Trust.

[6] Ministry of Agriculture, Fisheries and Food (1956), *Diets: Studies in Urban Household Diets, 1944-49*, second report of National Food Survey Committee, HMSO.

[7] Ministry of Agriculture, Fisheries and Food (1952), *Domestic Food Consumption and Expenditure, 1950*, annual report of the National Food Survey Committee, HMSO.

CHAPTER 3

How Nutritional Knowledge was Applied

Dorothy Hollingsworth

Although there was then still some uncertainty about the exact quantitative requirements for some nutrients "even in 1939 our knowledge was sufficiently detailed to enable the Government to evolve a most successful food policy during World War II" [1]. Thus, the outbreak of war in 1939 found Britain well fitted, given the political will, to apply the findings of the nutritional sciences to the job of feeding the population satisfactorily.

In the middle 1930s, the Health Committee of the League of Nations issued several important reports on nutrition. One of these, the 1936 report on the *Physiological Bases of Nutrition* [2], set out in quantitative terms the calorie and protein requirements of various categories of individual and made general recommendations about needs for minerals and vitamins, particularly in terms of the so-called protective foods. Concurrently, the Ministry of Health's Advisory Committee on Nutrition was considering the British diet. Its first Report, published in 1937, which incorporated the League of Nations recommendations, showed how that should be improved [3]. The Committee emphasised the need for increased consumption of safe milk by mothers, children and adolescents and expressed the hope that "the primary objective of the State will be to ensure that a supply of safe milk ... is brought within the purchasing power of the poorest". It thought that the national consumption of fruit and vegetables was below requirement for optimal nutrition and that potato consumption should be increased to replace "some of the sugar and highly milled cereals in ordinary diets".

Nutritional aspects of the food position

J C Drummond (Professor of Biochemistry at University College, London) was seconded to the Ministry of Food in the autumn of 1939 and appointed Scientific Adviser on 1 February 1940. Almost immediately he submitted a memorandum 'on certain nutritional aspects of the food position'.

He reviewed the pre-war food situation and the probable effects on it of wartime restrictions, particularly for the poor. He stressed the need for bread of high nutritive value, for increased consumption of potatoes, oatmeal, cheese and green vegetables, for supplying not less than one pint of milk a day for expectant and nursing mothers and all children up to the age of 15, and for fortifying all margarine with vitamins A and D. He aimed from the start not only to maintain but to improve the nutritional value of the diet. In May 1940, the Ministry of Food's import programme for the second year of war was produced and to it was appended a survey of wartime nutrition in which were set out in detailed and quantitiative form what were in effect Drummond's views on the type of nutritional strategy the Ministry should adopt [see 4]. The survey contained estimates of the nutritional requirements of the population and showed that the pre-war national food supply had been adequate in energy-rich foods but short in protective foods, particularly those supplying calcium, vitamin A and thiamin. The survey reviewed the dietary changes that occurred during the First World War, particularly the deterioration in the supply of minerals and vitamins for vulnerable groups of people, and indicated how this danger could be averted in the Second World War. The nutritional value of expected home production of food in 1940-41 was calculated. The import programme was considered and the resulting total food supply was assessed. As a result, recommendations were made for;

- increasing the supply of thiamin either by raising the extraction rate of flour or by fortifying white flour with synthetic thiamin;

- expanding home production of milk and vegetables, including potatoes;

- increasing imports of cheese, dried and condensed milks, canned fatty fish and pulses;

- importing vitamin A and D concentrates to add to margarine;

- reducing imports of fruits (other than oranges), nuts and eggs-in-shell (as being wasteful of shipping).

The impossibility of reducing supplies of energy-rich foods without impairing health was emphasised.

Most of these proposals became part of the Government's food policy and the rationing system, the details of which were kept under constant review, took into account the nutritional aspects of food policy. The Wartime Food Survey was one of the means of review. For example, I remember being asked by Drummond what would be the effect on the nutritional value of the working-class diet of the reduction of one ounce in the weekly cheese ration. Another means of review was the Body Weight Survey, mentioned below.

Assessing nutritional value

I was appointed to the Ministry's Statistics and Intelligence Division in Colwyn Bay in May 1941 as a dietetic statistician with the task of assessing the nutritional value of the diet of the families participating in the Wartime Food Survey. At that time there was no way to do this because no table of food composition had been compiled to fit the foods recorded.

At about the same time, the Accessory Food Factors (i.e. vitamins) Committee of the Medical Research Council undertook the responsibility of compiling data which were first published in 1945 under the title *Nutritive Values of Wartime Foods* [5]. The need for this compilation was set out in the introduction to the publication as follows:-

" (i) Values for the composition of many foodstuffs consumed in wartime were not available in existing tables; the differences between the values for wartime and peacetime foods are often great.

(ii) In Britain, values for the vitamins in foods have not previously been scrutinised and tabulated in a form suitable for use in evaluating dietary data.

(iii) Dietary surveys of the population, which are being carried out by the Ministry of Food and the Ministry of Health, have created a demand for food tables, giving, for raw foods, values for the proteins, fats and carbohydrates, and for the relatively small number of minerals and vitamins most likely to be deficient in the human diet."

Many people were consulted in the preparation of the new tables. A list of the institutions consulted is given in the publication. There was much argument, particularly about the method of converting grams of carbohydrate, protein and fat into energy value, and also that for converting grams of ß-carotene into vitamin A potency.

Although not published until 1945, the tables were available in draft form for use in the Ministry of Food, as soon as they were prepared. They gave values for the composition of raw foods per 100g in terms of 'edible portion' and 'as purchased' and 'per ounce as purchased'. The 'as purchased' figures made allowance for the inedible parts of foods, such as bones and the outside leaves and skins of vegetables, but not for the amount of edible food wasted in the kitchen or at table. Much of my early time in the Ministry was devoted to trying to assess wastage, mainly from the results of the Ministry of Health's *Precise Dietary Survey*, then recently completed but never published, in which wastage of edible food in the home was, at least, partially measured.

My job in Colwyn Bay was to make a table of food composition for application by the Ministry's Hollerith machines direct to the amounts of foods purchased. This required regular discussion with Ministry of Health officials and members of the Scientific Adviser's Division of the Ministry of Food, all of whom worked in London. This was of great personal benefit to me, a very young scientist, as it gave me the opportunity to get to know personally all the scientists in Britain who were contributing to the then new and experimental matter of calculating the nutritional value of the wartime diet.

The National Food Survey Committee, which was appointed in 1948, published its first report in 1951 [6]. It contained estimates of the energy value and nutrient composition of the urban working-class diet between 1940 and 1949, but no assessment of the nutritional adequacy of those diets, because no agreed standards of nutritional requirements of individuals were then available.

Recommended nutritional requirements

The first comprehensive recommendations for nutritional requirements were those of the League of Nations [2]. In 1941, the Food and Nutrition Board of the National Research Council of the USA made recommendations for 'dietary allowances', which they regarded as tentative. Soon after his appointment, Drummond compiled a table of nutritional requirements for use by the Ministry of Food in planning food supplies. It was based on the 1941 recommendations from the USA.

In 1950, the Committee on Nutrition of the British Medical Association (BMA) published its report [7], which included recommendations for nutritional requirements, based on an extensive review of the literature and on the observed effects of food shortage during wartime. As stated in the BMA report "In dealing with *nutritional needs* the Committees took only conditions of health into account. It admits that there may be exceptional requirements for individuals in various groups and that available estimates lack precision, but after reviewing the extensive literature of the subject it believes that the needs of representative individuals in each group are met by the figures given".

The BMA recommendations were adopted as soon as they were published to estimate what was termed, in the first annual report of the National Food Survey Committee published in 1952 [8], the 'adequacy of the diet'. Some of the difficulties encountered in making these estimates are discussed in the sections of that report on the diets of families of different social class and of different size in the following way:-

" Requirements are affected by age, sex and occupation and although the Survey records include details of each attribute, nutrient requirement scales are drawn up only in relation to age, sex and degree of activity, that is whether the work is light or heavy. Information on the degree of activity of different occupations is scanty and the allocation of occupations to the nutrient requirement categories has in consequence been largely arbitrary. The degree of activity in leisure-time pursuits is not known.

"A further difficulty arises from the lack of information on the nutritive value of meals eaten outside the home. To meet this problem, the appropriate level of requirements has been reduced by the proportion that the number of outside meals (weighted according to type) bears to the total number of meals normally taken at home.

Finally, many of the scales of nutrient requirements in common use, being based directly on the physiological requirements of the individual, relate to the food as eaten".

The report then explained that the inedible parts of food and the cooking losses of thiamin and vitamin C are allowed for in the Survey table of food composition and that 10 per cent is deducted from all estimates of consumption as "an arbitrary allowance for wastage in the kitchen and on the plate, for spoilage and for food fed to domestic pets", though it was recognised that for many nutrients this was probably too high.

The first comparisons of records of consumption with estimates of requirements calculated in this way for social classes and families of different size were published in the first NFS annual report [8]. I remember being well satisfied when the resulting percentages turned out to be reasonable. For example, the diet for *all households* was estimated to be 101 per cent of the BMA recommendations for energy value, compared with 98 per cent for old age pensioner families, 109 per cent for those with one child and 96 per cent for those containing both adolescents and children.

If the percentages fell below 100, concern was often expressed, sometimes by politicians. I remember, for example, being summoned by the Parliamentary Secretary, then Charles Hill, to justify the use of the 10 per cent wastage reduction for calcium. Concern about low values, particularly for protein and calcium in large families, began to be expressed in the late 1950s, and a special Panel of the Ministry of Health's Committee on Medical and Nutritional Aspects of Food Policy was appointed to consider the problem. It advised in 1960 [9] that "we need not be unduly perturbed when there is evidence that the intake of particular nutrients by certain sections of the community is somewhat less than the recommended allowance. If, however, there is a fall to 80-85 per cent of the allowance recommended by the BMA Committee this should be regarded as a signal for "watchful concern", words that became something of a catchphrase among those who worked on the Survey results. It also recommended that comparisons of estimates of intake with need should be "interpreted with caution" and explained that it was an "obviously inadmissable interpretation" to "conclude that, because the percentages are below 100, malnutrition must be widespread". Later, the Ministry of Health appointed a Panel to review the BMA recommendations. That Panel, reporting in 1969 recommended substantially smaller intakes of protein and calcium [10].

A table in the 1967 NFS annual report [11] shows the result of applying the new recommendations. For protein in all households the former 106 per cent would become 128 per cent and in larger families 93 per cent would become 115 per cent. The corresponding figures for calcium, were, respectively, 110 per cent, 191 per cent, 92 per cent and 166 per cent. There were smaller changes for other nutrients while the energy percentages remained almost as originally calculated. The new DHSS recommendations were adopted for the 1968 NFS annual report [12] and, with subsequent slight revisions, are still in use. This short disgression illustrates the kind of vicissitude we met in the Survey's early years.

The methods used to calculate the nutritional value of the household diet and its adequacy were novel at the time of adoption. They were part of what has turned out to be a successful experiment. Despite adjustments to accommodate new knowledge they are still essentially as they were at the outset. Such constancy confirms the soundness of the original concepts.

The Body Weight Survey

Between 1943 and 1949, a survey of the body weight of the adult population of Great Britain aged 25 to 54 years was made for the Ministry of Food with the aim of providing an independent check on the adequacy of the food supply [13]. On certain broad assumptions a fall in body weight would have been a warning that food supplies were inadequate. No gross changes were found.

Continuous records were obtained for male and female industrial workers in small firms and for working-class housewives who spent most of their time looking after their homes. Average changes in weight, based on 3,000 to 4,500 individuals, are shown by quarters from April 1943 to October 1949 in Figures 3.1 and 3.2.

Figure 3.1
Changes in weight of adult males, 1943-49

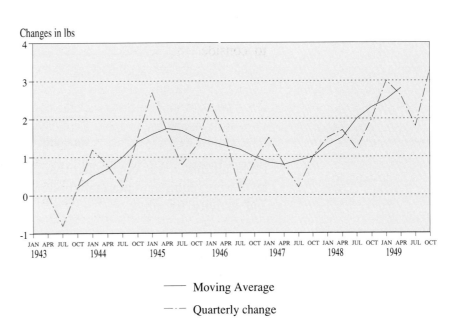

—— Moving Average

— ·— Quarterly change

Figure 3.2
Changes in weight
of adult females,
1943-49

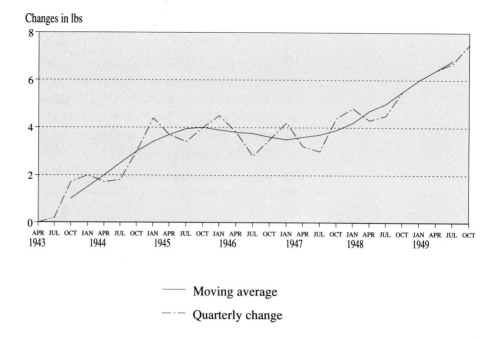

Changes in lbs

—— Moving average

—·— Quarterly change

Figure 3.3 shows changes in the calorie value of working-class household food consumption recorded by the Wartime Food Survey for 20,000 to 30,000 individuals for the same quarters. There was independent evidence that the growth rates of children were retarded during the years when the body weights of adults fell.

Figure 3.3
Changes in energy
value for working
class diets, 1943-49

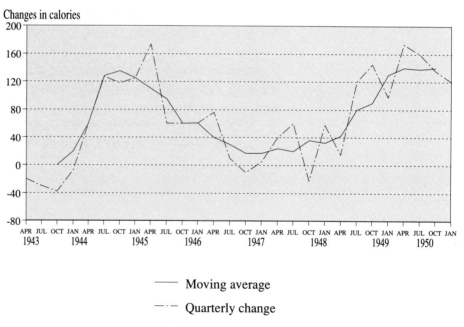

Changes in calories

—— Moving average

—·— Quarterly change

From all this it was concluded that 2,900 - 3,000 kcal/day at the retail level were required to maintain body weight of adults, growth in children and activity for all.

I acknowledge, with gratitude, the scientific opportunities my work for the National Food Survey gave me and the present need to remember some of my early scientific experiences. Though the Survey may change, I hope it will provide future workers with the sort of stimulus I enjoyed during its experimental years.

REFERENCES

[1] Agricultural Research Council / Medical Research Council (1974), *Food and Nutrition Research*, report of Committee on Food and Nutrition Research, HMSO.

[2] League of Nations (1937), *Physiological Bases of Nutrition,* Report of the Technical Commission of the Health Committee, New York.

[3] Ministry of Health (1937), *First Report of Advisory Committee on Nutrition,* HMSO.

[4] Drummond, J C and Wilbraham, A (1957), *The Englishman's Food,* 2nd edition, 449, Jonathan Cape, London.

[5] Medical Research Council (1945), *Nutritive Values of Wartime Foods,* War Memorandum No. 14, HMSO.

[6] Ministry of Food (1951), *The Urban Working-Class Household Diet, 1940 to 1949,* first report of the National Food Survey Committee, HMSO.

[7] British Medical Association (1950), *Report of the Committee on Nutrition,* London.

[8] Ministry of Food (1952), *Domestic Food Consumption and Expenditure, 1950,* annual report of the National Food Survey Committee, HMSO.

[9] Department of Health and Social Security (1960), *Report of Expert Panel on Requirements of Protein, Calcium and Other Nutrients,* Committee on Medical and Nutritional Aspects of Food Policy, HMSO.

[10] Department of Health and Social Security (1969), *Recommended Intakes of Nutrients for the United Kingdom,* Reports on Public Health and Medical Subjects, No 120, HMSO.

[11] Ministry of Agriculture, Fisheries and Food (1969), *Household Food Consumption and Expenditure, 1967,* annual report of the National Food Survey Committee, HMSO.

[12] Ministry of Agriculture, Fisheries and Food (1970), *Household Food Consumption and Expenditure, 1968,* annual report of the National Food Survey Committee, HMSO.

[13] Kemsley, W F F (1953), *Changes in Bodyweight 1943 to 1950,* Annals of Eugenics, Vol 18.

SECTION III

The National Food Survey
and the
National Diet

CHAPTER 4

The Consumption Revolution

Christopher Ritson and Richard Hutchins

Introduction

The choice of food made by individuals and households is influenced by a large range of factors including, for example, prices, incomes, tastes, social attitudes, desire for convenience, and so on. It is, however, extremely difficult to say how important each factor is in influencing any particular food purchase.

It may be more relevant to try to explain why one household purchases a large quantity, and another only a small quantity, of a particular good, by comparing differences in the households. The explanation might lie, for example, in income differences, social background, price advantage, a food allergy or a host of other factors. Similarly it may be possible to explain why average levels of consumption of different foods change over time among the population as a whole. An understanding of the causes of changes in average levels of food consumption over time, and variations within the population, is of great interest to nutritionists, policy makers and the food industry. The National Food Survey (NFS) provides an invaluable source of data of relevance to these questions.

The past decade has seen substantial changes in patterns of food consumption in the United Kingdom and, if anything, the pace of change is accelerating. The central thesis of this paper is that, unlike earlier periods of rapid developments in food consumption, the major trends we are now experiencing are primarily the result of fundamental changes in the attitudes and social behaviour of British households. That is what is meant by the 'Consumption Revolution'.

Phases in the evolution of food consumption in the UK

In order to illustrate this point, Figure 4.1 provides a very simplified interpretation of the factors influencing changing patterns of food consumption during the life of the NFS. The period has been divided into five overlapping phases noting, for each phase, what we believe to have been the dominant factor influencing developments in food choice.

The first period has been labelled 'wartime austerity and rationing'. Individual food choice was largely *imposed* by availability, the consequences of which for the national diet were explored earlier. During the second phase, the end to rationing and more plentiful supplies allowed British households to return to what would then have been regarded, under the constraint of prevailing incomes and prices, as *normal* diets.

Figure 4.1
Periods of changing food consumption

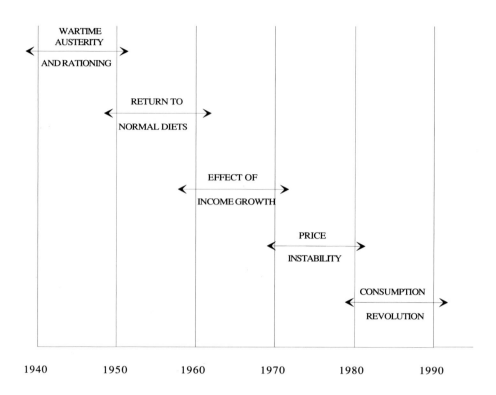

By the mid 1950s, the postwar rise in living standards was underway, and soon Mr Macmillan was claiming that "you have never had it so good". The effect for many households was to lift the income constraint gradually over a period of some 20 years, allowing consumers to move their diets in what they would regard as a preferred direction.

Examples of the main foods which would have been expected to experience increasing consumption as a consequence of rising personal incomes in the UK are given in Table 4.2. In contrast, for some foods, known as 'inferior goods', less is purchased as incomes rise.

	Consumption rises with income	Consumption falls with income
Table 4.2 Foods for which consumption was significantly affected by income growth	Cheese	Canned meat
	Canned salmon	Sausages
	Shell fish	Herrings
	Beef	Margarine
	Pork	Lard
	Chicken	Canned milk puddings
	Salad vegetables	Potatoes
	Salad oils	Dried pulses
	Frozen vegetables	Canned vegetables
	Fresh fruit	Tea
	Chocolate biscuits	White bread
	Brown and wholemeal bread	Oatmeal products
	Rice	
	Coffee	
	Ice-cream	

In some cases, the effects of income growth were probably quite substantial, leading perhaps to changes of 20-25 per cent over a twenty year period.

During the 1970s, however, prices became much more important as an influence on patterns of food consumption. A number of factors, for example the world commodities price boom, the adoption of the Common Agricultural Policy (CAP), the drought of 1975-76, and the food subsidy programme, caused extreme volatility in the retail prices of many food products. The effect of price instability on consumption of butter and margarine is shown in Figure 4.3.

Figure 4.3
Changing patterns of consumption of butter and margarine

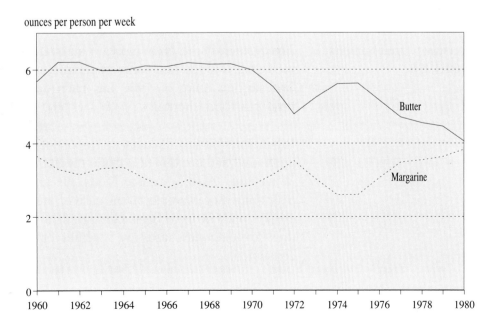

37

During the 1960s, butter consumption was relatively stable and margarine consumption was trending gently down, probably because of the income effect mentioned above. From 1970 to 1980 however, butter and margarine consumption become virtually mirror images of one another.

What happened was as follows:

(i)   The coincidence of dry Northern and Southern Hemisphere summers at the beginning of the decade led to a rise in world butter prices and, with most of butter imported at that time, UK retail prices rose. Butter consumption fell but this was largely replaced by increased household purchases of margarine.

(ii)   In the mid-Seventies, however, the world commodities boom raised vegetable oil prices, and thus margarine prices. Meanwhile, the British government introduced a food subsidy programme, which included butter, and international butter prices started to fall back to normal levels. Butter consumption therefore rose again at the expense of margarine consumption.

(iii)   Then World commodity prices fell as quickly as they had risen, and margarine prices also came down. Meanwhile, the application in the UK of minimum import prices under the CAP gradually took effect and butter prices rose. Once again there was a substantial shift within the yellow fats market, from butter to margarine.

By the end of the 1970s, the volatility of prices had subsided; world commodity prices had stabilised and British food prices had absorbed fully the affects of adopting the CAP. In fact, for most foods, prices then fell in real terms during the 1980s. Meanwhile the pace of income growth had slackened and the strength of the relationship between income and consumption seemed to lessen. Yet for many food products either the previous change in consumption was reversed or the pace of change accelerated.

Consumption changes: 1960-1980

The results of the NFS indicate significant changes in the patterns of food consumption and some of the major changes are described below. The starting point of 1960 has been taken because of the impact of post-war food shortages.

When interpreting changes in food consumption, the fact that meals purchased and consumed outside the home are excluded has to be taken in account. Also, for some foods, the form of the product has changed over time. For example, in the case of meat and vegetables, an increased proportion will have been purchased in a prepared and trimmed form, thus reducing purchases by weight but not necessarily the amount consumed.

Subject to these caveats, aggregate consumption for some food groups has remained remarkably stable. For instance, total meat consumption has been between 35 to 40 ounces per person per week for most of the 30 year period and, apart from the drought affected years of 1976 and 1977, total vegetable consumption has remained around 70 to 80 ounces per person per week. Fish consumption declined in the early part of the period reaching a low point in the mid 1970s. It has recovered almost to 1960 levels in recent years. Purchases of cereals and sugar have declined almost throughout the period although, in the case of the latter, this reflects a reduction in home preserving and jam making. For product groups such as milk and cream, fats and oils, beverages and eggs, a period of relative stability was succeeded by a period of decline. The only groups where consumption has shown a significant increase over the period are cheese and fruit.

In practice, a watershed appears to have occured for a number of food groups around 1975-80. Stable or rising consumption was replaced by decline or the pace of previous decline accelerated. With fish and fruit, decline and stability respectively were replaced by growth.

Within the food groups, changes are much more marked with considerable year to year fluctuations reflecting both economic and social effects. Even so, some distinct long term trends are discernable. For instance, as illustrated in Figure 4.4, consumption of beef and sheepmeat has declined although some of this decline has been offset by the dramatic rise in purchases of poultry. Added to which, expenditure but not volume, of meat products has increased substantially.

Figure 4.4
Consumption of meat

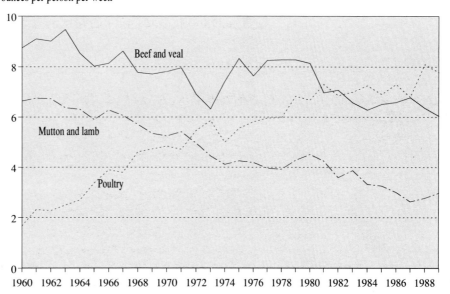

ounces per person per week

A particularly striking trend is the decline in consumption of whole milk since 1975 and the rapid increase in sales of low fat milks once they became readily available in the early 1980s (Figure 4.5).

Figure 4.5
Consumption of milks

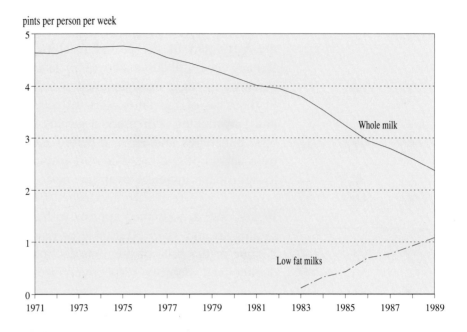

For fish, a fall in overall consumption was mainly due to the rapid decline in fresh fish sales between 1968 and 1975. Since then, fresh fish sales have stabilised and the growth in the frozen fish market has resulted in a recovery in total fish consumption.

In Figure 4.6, the data for the fats and oils market has been extended through the 1980s. During this latter period, butter consumption has plummeted and margarine and lard consumption have also joined the decline. These have been replaced in the diet to some extent by vegetable and salad oils and, in recent years, by low fat spreads.

Figure 4.6
Consumption of oils and fats

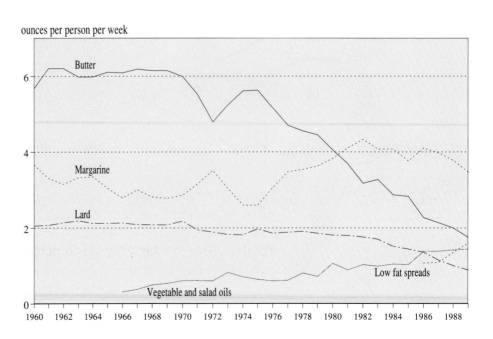

Among the vegetables, declining consumption of cabbage, cauliflower and brussels sprouts has only partially been offset by higher purchases of salad vegetables. Similarly, consumption of traditional root vegetables and of canned vegetables have tended to decline while purchases of frozen vegetables have increased.

A significant rise in consumption of fruit since the mid 1970s is partially accounted for by the very sharp rise in purchases of fruit juice and the increasing range of fruit available throughout the year. Apples, pears, citrus and bananas continue to account for the major proportion of fruit purchases.

For beverages, the modest growth in coffee sales has failed to offset the substantial fall in purchases of tea.

One of the most significant changes has been a decline in consumption of white bread which has only partially been offset by an increase for brown, wholemeal and wholewheat bread. The decline in consumption of cakes, which was very rapid between 1968 and 1978, appears to have halted and purchases of biscuits have been fairly stable in recent years. However, consumption of breakfast cereals has increased steadily and is more than twice the level of 30 years ago (Figure 4.7).

Figure 4.7
Consumption of cereal products

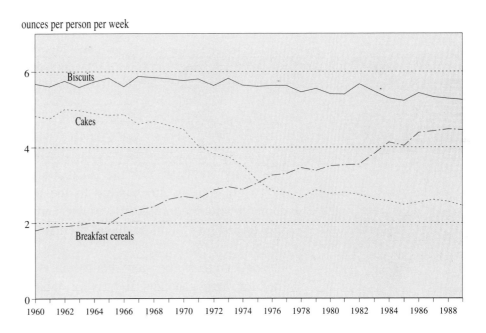

ounces per person per week

The underlying trend in demand

As already emphasised, food choice is influenced by a large range of factors. Information on some of these factors, such as prices paid and household income, are collected in the Survey. Analyses of these data make it possible to establish what proportion of past changes in purchases can be attributed to changes in prices and incomes. What is left, the residual - known as the 'underlying trend in demand' - is attributable to a large number of other economic and social factors such as consumer tastes and household characteristics. Professor Chesher analyses, in a later paper, the impact of household composition on the pattern of consumption but, for some purposes, it may arguably suffice to look at movements in underlying demand. In effect, to the extent that this shows what would have happened in the absence of changes in prices and incomes, underlying demand may provide a better guide to successful marketing than trends in actual consumption.

By way of illustration, Figure 4.8 shows purchases, price and demand trend for meat and meat products. The data are in the form of index numbers; that is, they are expressed as a percentage of the average values during the base period. It should be emphasised therefore that the graphs show relative trends and the absolute differences between the lines are not important.

Figure 4.8
Purchases, price and underlying trend for meat and meat products

Index: 1978-1983 average = 100

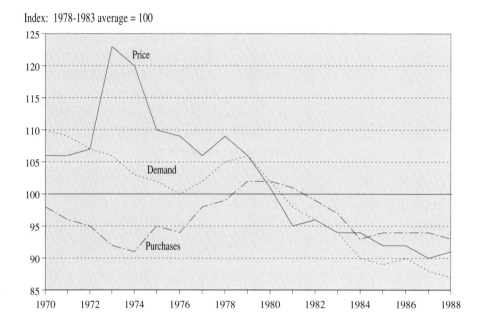

This graph indicates that the fluctuations in meat purchases during the 1970s are mainly attributable to the movement in price. Underlying demand remained relatively stable but, subsequently, both purchases and underlying demand have declined quite rapidly.

The data confirm the view that the period 1975-1980 represents a watershed for many products. Relatively stable demand is replaced by a strong positive or negative development and the underlying trend in demand begins to dominate the way patterns of food consumption are changing in the UK.

The long term changes in behaviour, and attributes which underlie trends in demand, are unlikely to cause average levels of consumption of different foods to fluctuate erratically - except in exceptional cases such as the recent food scares which affected purchases of eggs and beef. Thus, the year-on-year fluctuations in the demand trends are most probably the consequence of a mixture of sampling error and the failure to identify accurately the effect of price changes.

In an attempt to overcome this problem, simple linear trends were fitted to 155 foods or food groups for which data were available. A league table was drawn up ranking the products from those with the highest underlying trend in demand to those with the lowest. The 'top ten' are listed in Figure 4.9 below.

Figure 4.9
Products with highest growth in underlying demand

Food Code	Product	Annual Per Cent Change in Demand
171	Other fresh green vegetables (eg: spinach, broccoli)	+29
256	Wholewheat and wholemeal bread	+18
205	Frozen chips and other frozen convenience potato products	+13
148	All other fats (eg: low fat spreads)	+12
294	Frozen convenience cereal foods (eg. pastries and pizzas)	+11
202	Other vegetable products (inc. prepared salads)	+ 9
248	Fruit juices	+ 8
200	Crisps and other potato products, not frozen	+ 7
231	Other fresh fruit (eg: melons, pineapples and exotics)	+ 7
117	Shellfish	+ 6

The list makes interesting reading. Two features of 'star' products stand out; they seem to be associated either with convenience or healthy eating.

The bottom ten are given in Figure 4.10 below.

Figure 4.10
Products with largest fall in underlying demand

Food Code	Product	Annual Per Cent Change in Demand
105	Fresh white fish, unfilleted	-22
168	Fresh peas	-16
116	Processed fat fish, unfilleted	-15
227	Soft fresh fruit, other than grapes	-15
198	Instant potato	-10
51	Offals, other than liver	- 9
315	Baby foods, canned and bottled	-8
233/236	Canned and bottled fruit	- 8
199	Canned potatoes	- 7
103	Brussels sprouts	- 7

It should be emphasised that these reflect changes in underlying demand, not consumption. They attempt to indicate the extent to which underlying behaviour and attitudes of the population towards different foods are changing. In some cases the figures contradict market growth, or decline, if sales have been strongly affected by positive or negative price developments.

Factors affecting underlying demand

It was not the purpose of this paper to attempt a complete explanation of these underlying trends in demand. Some of the evidence lies outside the NFS, in market research data, and some of the subsequent papers explore aspects of the NFS which do contribute to an explanation. However, attention is drawn here to two factors which are of importance.

First, a number of changes within the household, particularly the increase in the number of working women and the breakdown of traditional meal patterns in the home, have led to a desire for foods which are easy to prepare, quick to cook, and which come in individual portions. This not only affects the obvious foods, such as frozen convenience products, but also, for example, the form in which meat is presented, eg, chops and mince rather than joints.

At Newcastle, a food diary study explored meal patterns within the household [1]. This revealed the astonishing degree to which fast food had taken over *within* the household. Some 94 per cent of meals involved less than 10 minutes preparation time, and 51 per cent no preparation time whatsoever. Some 61 per cent of all meals involved no cooking time and only 7 per cent more than 20 minutes cooking time.

The second factor is what is known as the 'vintage effect'. The stage in the family life cycle, characterised by the recorded age of the housewife in the NFS, provides one of the best explanations of differences in patterns of household consumption for some foods. The typical pattern, illustrated in Figure 4.11, is one of less than average consumption at early stages (young single people and young marrieds), rising to a peak when the housewife is in her fifties (the children have left the household and disposable income is high) and then declining towards the average for pensioner households.

Figure 4.11
Total food expenditure
by age of housewife

£ per person per week compared with national average

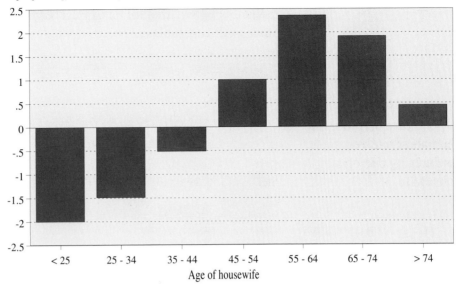

The consumption variations according to age can be attributed to two effects. First, the structure of the household (size, number of children, etc), proportion of meals eaten outside the home, and income of the household will be closely connected with the age of the housewife and this will influence patterns of consumption. Second, consumption habits are formed by children and young adults and they carry these habits through with them as they grow older. The latter, the 'vintage' effect, can clearly have a profound influence on which products display rising, and which declining, underlying trends in demand.

Figure 4.12 illustrates the vintage effect on purchases of mutton and lamb, where it is the 'older' households who spend above the average on the product.

Figure 4.12
Expenditure on
mutton and lamb
by age of housewife

Pence per person per week compared with national average

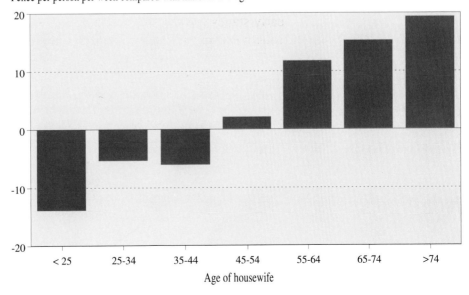

45

A different pattern emerges for processed vegetables and vegetable products, where the 'older' households depend less on frozen and processed vegetables.

Figure 4.13
Expenditure on processed vegetables and vegetable products by age of housewife

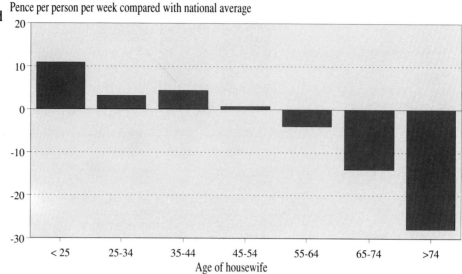

Pence per person per week compared with national average

Age of housewife

Conclusion

Thus the National Food Survey provides a wealth of information which enables historic patterns of food consumption to be explained and the future of the 'Consumption Revolution' to be predicted.

REFERENCES

[1] Gofton, L R and Marshall, D (1989), *A Comprehensive Scientific Study of the Behavioural Variables Affecting Acceptability of Fish Products as a Basis for Determining Options in Fish Utilisation Research and Development at Torry Research Station,* unpublished report for the Ministry of Agriculture, Fisheries and Food.

CHAPTER 5

The Changing Household Diet

David Buss

Introduction

The continuity of the National Food Survey (NFS) means that it is possible to determine exactly how the British household diet has changed over the past 50 years, and be sure that the results are internally consistent. This has enormous social as well as nutritional and economic value, and is not possible in any other country. The database is, however, very large; it covers 400,000 households, and represents the diets of 1¼ million people over that time - or 25,000 people-years of records. Furthermore, since the survey became truly national in 1950, each annual report has given details of foods and their cost and nutritional value in nine regions, half-a-dozen social classes or income bands and about ten different breakdowns of household composition. So even without counting the analyses by age of housewife, by urbanisation, housing tenure, freezer-ownership or the numerous special analyses, there have been more than 25 detailed tables per year for 40 years.

It is possible to show only a tiny fraction of this information and this paper focuses particularly on foods of current nutritional interest. These include foods low in fats, in contrast to the foods of particular concern in earlier years. In the 1940s, for example, it was much more important to increase the fat content of the diet, for fat was in short supply and people were complaining [1]. Indeed, even as late as 1966 the Department of Education and Science set nutritional standards which required a *minimum* of 1.15 ounces of fat in every school meal, and these remained in force until 1975 [2].

Trends in fat and carbohydrate

Intakes of fat and carbohydrate are often considered in terms of the proportion of the dietary energy that they provide, as well as the absolute amounts eaten. In 1984, a Department of Health committee recommended that the proportion of energy derived from fat should not exceed 35 per cent when the NFS showed it to be 42 per cent [3]. Figure 5.1 shows that it last provided this amount as long ago as 1947. At that time, both the absolute intake of fat and the contributions made by meat, fats, dairy products and other foods were similar to those made now. However, this fat was far more saturated, for there was much more fat on beef and lamb, and suet and hard margarines were very important fats.

Figure 5.1
Percentage of energy
from carbohydrate,
fat and protein

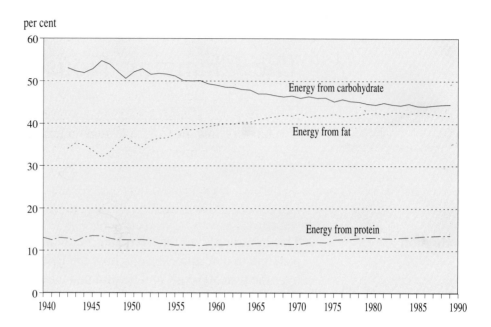

Although fat intakes subsequently rose to between 4.00 and 4.25 ounces/day in the 1960s, as people finally had ready access to it, the reason for the lower proportion of energy from fat during and after the war was the much larger amount of carbohydrate eaten at that time. In 1947, total carbohydrate intakes were around 11.30 ounces/day (providing 55 per cent of the energy) and were mainly starch. When rationing ended, people ate more sugar as well as more fat, and packet sugar purchases rose from about 1.25 ounces/day during the war to 2.65 ounces/day in 1958. They then dropped steadily until they are now only 0.90 ounces/day. Although more sugar may be eaten now in commercial cakes, biscuits, etc, because domestic home baking, fruit bottling and jam making have declined, total sugar supplies in the country have also decreased markedly during this time [4].

As fat and sugar purchases increased, starch declined - but it has continued to decline ever since, even though sugar (and fat) have also fallen. So total energy intakes are now much lower, and the carbohydrate intake in 1989 was estimated at only 8.10 ounces/day.

The British diet from 1940 to 1989

The broad pattern of the British diet during the past 50 years is shown in Figure 5.2. Its consistency is remarkable, considering all the social and economic changes during that time, including changes in the age and ethnic structure of the population, smaller families, changes in working patterns including the increase in working women, the switch from staples to pre-prepared foods such as frozen foods and ready-meals and to foreign foods, the use of freezers and microwaves in place of traditional cooking, inflation, and EEC entry. The British diet has in fact, remained just that - a British diet - and is still recognisably different from a French diet, a German diet, a Scandinavian diet or an Italian diet. It is still based to a considerable extent on bread, milk, meat and potatoes; is relatively low in fruit and vegetables; and, among alcoholic drinks, beer is drunk rather than wine. These are the foods that grow well in a northern grassland climate. What has happened, though, is that there have been greater changes within each of these broad food types. For instance, traditional vegetables such as swedes, parsnips and brussels sprouts have been superceded by mushrooms and salad vegetables. An over-simplification of the changes might be that there has been a switch from traditional roast beef, roast potatoes and cabbage in the middle of the day, to microwaved chicken, frozen chips, and courgettes as an evening snack.

Figure 5.2
Trends in consumption of major food groups

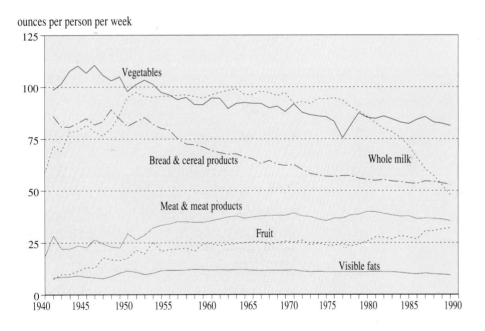

ounces per person per week

(a) **Milk:** The one food in Figure 5.2 that has been rather less constant is milk. During the war successful efforts were made to increase milk supplies and to get children in particular to drink it because of its high nutritional value. Consumption then remained steady until the mid 1970s, but *whole* milk consumption has almost halved since then. This fall began before the recent denigration of its fat content, so other factors must have played a part in this - including the increased popularity of other drinks and especially soft drinks. But, since 1984, skimmed and semi-skimmed milks have offset most of the decline.

(b) Fats: Although total consumption of fats remained steady at around 12.00 ounces/week from the mid 1950s to the early 1970s and are still around 9.50 ounces/week, there have been some major changes within that (Figure 5.3). The increase after the nadir in 1947 was mainly in the sought-after butter. However, from 1955 to about 1985, butter and margarine oscillated as alternatives. After 1975, the increase in margarine was essentially in the soft types that spread straight from the fridge. The recent concern about saturated fat has led to butter consumption dropping until it is now only at a quarter of its 1970 level, and to marked increases in vegetable oils and most recently to reduced-fat spreads.

Figure 5.3
Trends in consumption of visible fats

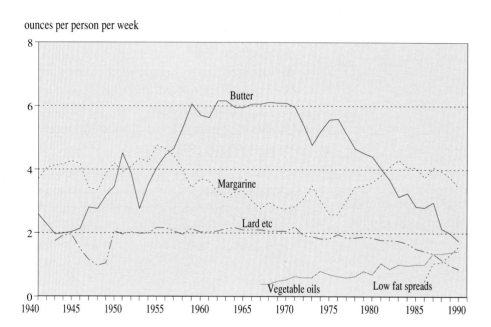

(c) Meat: Consumption of beef, lamb and pigmeat all rose sharply in the early 1950s, but since then the main changes have been the steady decline in lamb and the seemingly inexorable rise in poultry consumption (Figure 5.4). Poultry is now more important than beef, yet 40 years ago chicken was essentially a once-a-year treat at Christmas. Among meat products, one of the more important changes has been the increasing popularity of frozen products and, more recently, of exotic products such as paté, parallelling the changes that have occurred with vegetables and fruit.

Figure 5.4
Trends in consumption
of major meats

ounces per person per week

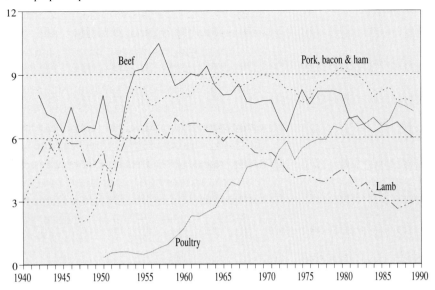

(d) Breads: Perhaps the most dramatic change during the whole of the past 50 years has been the sudden reversion from 'national bread' to white bread as soon as the latter was allowed to be made again, as shown in Figure 5.5. Although the consumption of wholemeal bread increased from 1978 until 1986 with the interest in fibre (and perhaps just as important, its improved texture), this did not reverse the long-term decline in white bread consumption in the home. Household bread consumption is thus lower than it has ever been in this country.

Figure 5.5
Trends in consumption
of bread

ounces per person per week

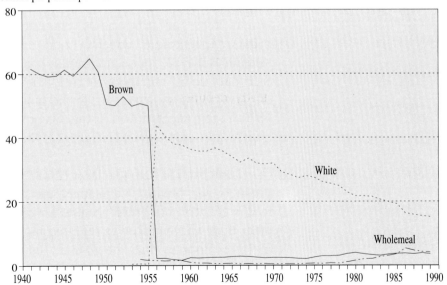

51

Some nutritional consequences

It has been possible to evaluate changes in certain nutrients every year from 1940 to the present. These are energy, total protein and animal and vegetable protein, calcium and iron, three B-vitamins (thiamin, riboflavin and niacin), vitamin C, and vitamin D. Vitamin A was added in 1942 and fat in 1943, but carbohydrate was not formally shown in the Survey until the 1951 annual report. These minerals and vitamins were the ones used for assessing Wartime nutrition policies, because American (and League of Nations) recommendations were available for these [5]. From 1950, however, the minerals and vitamins mentioned above could be compared with new British Medical Association recommendations [6], and there have subsequently been new yardsticks for these same nutrients from the Department of Health and Social Security in 1969 [7] and 1979 [8]. These yardsticks do not necessarily stay constant, as indicated in Table 5.6.

Table 5.6
Recommended intakes of selected nutrients in Britain during the past 50 years

per day for adult males

	Wartime	BMA 1950	DHSS 1969	DHSS 1979
Calcium (mg)	800	800	500	500
Vitamin C (mg)	75	20	30	30
Vitamin D (µg)	10	0	2.5	0

The Ministry's Nutrition Branch annually updates the factors used for assessing the nutritional value of each food, and has considerably extended the number of nutrients assessed, too. Over the past 15 years, national intakes of most other nutrients have been assessed including individual amino acids and fatty acids, cholesterol, fibre fractions, individual sugars, magnesium, copper, zinc, sodium, potassium, phosphorus, vitamin B6, B12, folic acid, biotin, pantothenic acid and vitamin E.[1] In fact, fatty acids, and more recently sodium, total fibre and total sugars, are now routinely evaluated in the quarterly and annual reports of the NFS. In this paper, however, there is only space to consider two nutrients briefly and calcium and vitamin C have been chosen.

(a) Calcium: The main sources of calcium in the British diet are dairy products and bread. Vegetables are still comparatively unimportant in this country, but bread became a major contributor when most flour, other than wholemeal, was required by law to be fortified with calcium in 1943. Prior to that, the intake did not meet the Wartime recommendation of 800 mg per day, but it then rose to 855 mg per day, and remained between 1000 and 1050 mg per day from 1948 to 1977.

1   See References [9, 10, 11, 12, 13, 14, 15, 16, 17, 18]

The subsequent decline in milk consumption (but not in other dairy products such as cheese and the increasingly popular yogurt), together with the continuing decline in fortified white bread, has led to a fall in calcium intakes to 840 mg per day in 1989. Although this intake is still high compared with most other countries where less milk is drunk and flour is not fortified, it demonstrates how certain restrictions in the diet, although possibly undertaken for health reasons, can lead to other undesirable nutritional consequences.

(b) Vitamin C: This is derived from fruit and vegetables. Potatoes were plentiful during the War but fruit was not. The intake of vitamin C was initially recorded as between 75 and 100 mg per day during the War, but this was without allowance for inevitable cooking losses. After adjustment, the intake in 1942 becomes only 38 mg (much less than the target), and vegetables other than potatoes contributed only 10 mg (26 per cent of the total) and fruit 7 mg (18 per cent). The subsequent rise in consumption of fruit, and most recently in fruit juices, has offset a decline from potatoes (Figure 5.7). Throughout the 1980s, vitamin C intakes have been close to 60 mg per day with fruit and fruit juices now contributing 25 mg per person per day, or 46 per cent of the total intake in 1989.

Figure 5.7
Trends in consumption of vegetables

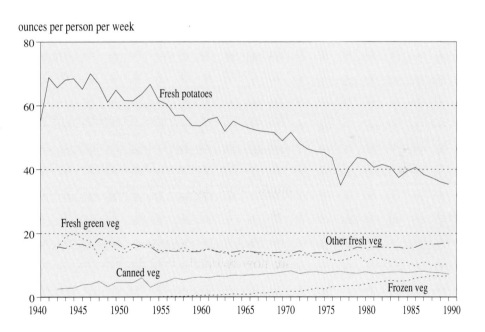

Conclusion

The changes in the British diet over the past 50 years have brought fat and sugar intakes back to their Wartime levels. Starch, however, has declined markedly so that for the past 25 years, 42 per cent of the dietary energy has been derived from fat. Some minerals and vitamins have increased while others have declined but, as life expectancy has increased substantially both for men and for women since the 1940s, our diet is probably better now than it has ever been.

REFERENCES

[1] Ministry of Food (1951), *The Urban Working Class Household Diet 1940 to 1949,* first report of the National Food Survey Committee, HMSO.

[2] Department of Education Science (1966), *The School Meals Service: The Nutritional Standard of School Dinners,* Science Circular 3/66.

[3] Department of Health and Social Security (1984), *Diet and Cardiovascular Disease,* report of the Committee on Medical Aspects of Food Policy, HMSO.

[4] Department of Health (1989), *Dietary Sugar and Human Disease,* HMSO.

[5] Hollingsworth, D F (1984), *Dietary Standards,* in Present Knowledge in Nutrition (5th Edition), The Nutrition Foundation, Washington D.C.

[6] British Medical Association (1950), *Report of the Committee on Nutrition,* London.

[7] Department of Health and Social Security (1969), *Recommended Intakes of Nutrients for the United Kingdom,* Reports on Public Health and Medical Subjects, No 120, HMSO.

[8] Department of Health and Social Security (1979), *Recommended Daily Amount of Food Energy and Nutrients for Groups of People in the United Kingdom,* HMSO.

[9] Buss, D H and Ruck, N F (1977), *The Amino Acid Pattern of the British Diet,* Human Nutrition, Vol 31.

[10] Bull, N L, Day, M J L, Burt, R and Buss, D H (1983), *Individual Fatty Acids in the British Household Food Supply,* Human Nutrition; Applied Nutrition Vol 37A.

[11] Spring, J A, Robertson, J and Buss, D H (1978), *The Cholesterol Content of Household Diets in Britain,* Proceedings of Nutrition Society, Vol 37.

[12] Robertson, J (1972), *Changes in the Fibre Content of the British Diet,* Nature, Vol 238, 290; Southgate, D A T, Bingham, S and Robertson, J, (1987) *Dietary Fibre in the British Diet,* Nature, Vol 274; Wenlock, R W, Buss, D H and Agater, I B (1984), *New Entrants of Fibre in the Diet in Britain,* British Medical Journal, Vol 288.

[13] Lewis, J and Buss, D H (1990), *Intakes of Individual Sugars in Britain,* Proceeding of Nutrition Society, Vol 49, 58A.

[14] Spring, J A, Robertson, J and Buss, D H (1979), *Trace Nutrients 3. Magnesium, Copper, Zinc, Vitamin B6, Vitamin B12 and Folic Acid in the British Household Food Supply,* British Journal of Nutrition, Vol 41; Lewis, J and Buss, D H (1988), *Trace Nutrients 5. Minerals and Vitamins in the British Household Food Supply,* British Journal of Nutrition Vol 60.

[15] Bull, N L and Buss, D H (1980), *Contributions of Foods to Sodium Intakes,* Proceeding of Nutrition Society, Vol 39, 30A.

[16] Bull, N L and Buss, D H (1980), *Contributions of Foods to Potassium Intakes,* Proceeding of Nutrition Society, Vol 39, 31A.

[17] Gilbert, L, Wenlock, R W and Buss, D H (1985), *Phosphorus in the British Household Food Supply,* Human Nutrition; Applied Nutrition Vol 39A.

[18] Buss, N L and Buss, D H (1982), *Biotin, Pantothenic Acid and Vitamin E,* Journal of Human Nutrition, Vol 36A.

CHAPTER 6

Household Composition and Household Food Purchases

Andrew Chesher

Introduction

The National Food Survey (NFS) is a unique source of information on food purchasing and indirectly on food consumption. Much diverse information can be extracted from it. By comparing purchases over time and relating changes in amounts purchased to changes in relative prices, demand equations can be estimated. By comparing the many thousands of households captured in a year's survey work, differences in household characteristics can be related to differences in food purchases and acquisitions. The NFS obtains information from a very wide variety of households. One respect in which they vary greatly is in their composition. This paper provides two examples of what can be obtained from the NFS regarding the impact of household composition on household food acquisition and consumption.

This type of analysis is of value to both government and industry. From the government's point of view, it is helpful to know how households of different types react to changes in prices and incomes. These matters become particularly relevant when proposals relating to such issues as taxes and subsidies are under consideration in the European Community (EC), when the provision of income supplements to poor households is being considered and for many other policy proposals. From the viewpoint of food manufacturers and retailers the analysis provides insight into the market for foods. It facilitates the prediction of demand for foods of different types as one passes from regions with different representations of household types. By keeping track of demographic changes it allows the prediction of changes in future demand.

Household composition has a substantial effect on household food consumption and this has long been recognised in analyses of the NFS data. Each year tables in the annual report of the NFS Committee [1] show how food acquisitions and the nutrients obtained from them vary across households classified by household composition type. Some care is required in analysing data of this sort because household composition tends to be correlated with other household characteristics such as income.

This is evident even in the very earliest reports of the Survey. For example, in the 1950 report of the NFS Committee [2], attention is drawn to the higher per capita consumption of milk by childless couples than by couples with four or more children even though the latter had the benefit of subsidised milk.

Similar higher rates of consumption by childless couples were observed for many other foods. It is likely that these are due to the relatively higher per capita income of childless couples and the other pressing demands made by children on household budgets. To get useful information on the effect of household composition it is essential to control for the effect of household income. In the next section some results concerning the effect of household composition and income on food expenditure obtained using the most recent survey data are presented. They demonstrate what can be drawn out from the data. Hopefully they will encourage further research.

The final section of this paper extends this analysis to the intake of nutrients. Here it emerges that the impact of income is far less important. However the impact of household composition is much more marked. This final section draws on results from a recent report [3] to show how nutrient consumptions of individuals of different types can be estimated, even though the NFS records only expenditures at the household level and not consumption of foods either by households or individuals. Of particular interest is the fact that the continuity of the NFS enables time series of nutrient consumption estimates to be constructed for different types of household member. This allows us to see whether young and old, males and females have been moving towards healthier diets or whether particular groups have fallen behind across all trends.

Household composition and food expenditure

Cross classification of households gives some insight into the impact of household composition on food expenditures but in considering very fine cross classifications, sampling variation starts to become intrusive. Another difficulty with cross classifications is that it is difficult to control for variations in income which, as noted above, may mask household composition effects. One way around these problems is to specify a model for household food expenditure that embodies the effect of household composition and income and to estimate the model's parameters using the NFS data. That is the approach adopted here.

How should income appear in such a model? Figure 6.1 shows survey week expenditure on food and net of tax weekly household income plotted against each other for 4,839 households observed in the 1989 NFS recording net income above £40 per week. A number of features are evident.

First there is clearly a great deal of variation in both food expenditure and in income. Variation in income indicates that the survey captures a wide range of households and it allows us to derive accurate estimates of the effect of income on food expenditure.

It would be better if there were less variation in food expenditure but what we see in Figure 6.1 is an accurate reflection of the variability in food expenditure and we must live with it. This variability arises first because households do differ from one another in the amount they spend on average on food and second because the amount they spend varies through time and the NFS captures just one week of their food purchasing experience.

Figure 6.1
Food expenditure and household income for 1989 NFS households

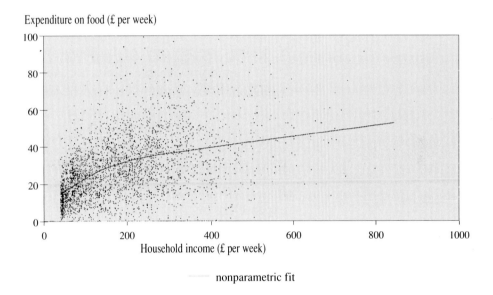

nonparametric fit

The week that a household is in the NFS may coincide with a week when it shops for food hardly at all. Such observations are compensated by records from households for which the Survey week coincides with an extensive shopping expedition. Consequently, though the NFS data are quite scattered, the averages the NFS produces are good estimates of average rates of household food expenditure and of consumption from household supplies.

A second notable feature of Figure 6.1 is that the relationship between food expenditure and income seems to be non-linear. The line passing through the scatter plot is a flexible function fitted using non-parametric methods[1]. It suggests that food expenditure increases with income but at a slower rate the higher income becomes.

1   The procedure used is the smoothing procedure described by Cleveland [4] as implemented in Becker, Chambers and Wilks' programme New S [5]. The smoothing procedure was not iterated to reduce the impact of 'outliers' because it is intended to pick up the variation in average expenditure with income and, in the presence of skewed data, iterating hinders this.

A widely used model for household expenditures, capable of capturing this feature, is the Working-Leser relationship [6,7] in which the share of total expenditure spent on a food, or group of foods, is written as a linear function of the logarithm of income. This model has been found to provide a good fit to expenditure data and it is easy to interpret. It was recently taken up as the basic expenditure - total outlay relationship in the Almost Ideal Demand model [8]. The basic form of the Working-Leser model is:

$$S_i = \frac{e_i}{x} = \alpha_i + \beta_i \log(x) + \varepsilon_i \qquad [A]$$

where:
S_i is the share of total expenditure on food i
e_i denotes survey week expenditure on food i
x denotes weekly net of tax household income
ε_i is a random variable capturing, across households and across time, variation in expenditure not associated with household income.

The parameters α_i and β_i will vary from food to food and it is these we wish estimate. If β_i were zero then food expenditure would be proportional to income. However Figure 6.1 strongly suggests that this is not the case and further that β is less than zero, at least for expenditure on 'all food'.

In Figure 6.2, the data of Figure 6.1 are replotted, this time expressing food expenditure as a proportion of income and using log income instead of income on the horizontal axis. If the Working-Leser model is going to be useful here, then in this form the data should be scattered around a straight line[2]. This does seem to be the case.

Two lines are superimposed on the scatter plot in Figure 6.2. The solid line is a flexible function fitted to the data as in Figure 6.1 and is designed to track the relationship between average food share and log income. The path it follows is remarkably close to a straight line. For reference, the dotted line is the result of fitting a straight line to the data by ordinary least squares.

Figure 6.2 suggests that the Working-Leser equation does a good job of picking up the functional form of the 'all food' Engel curve. It is used in the remainder of this section. Figure 6.2 also reveals how substantially the variance of the food share reduces as we pass to higher income households.

---

2 Because this graphical analysis does not control for variation in household composition it can only be regarded as indicative.

Figure 6.2

Food share and household income for 1989 NFS households

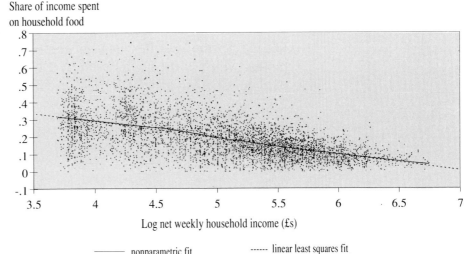

This leads us to use robust standard errors[3] when reporting measures of the accuracy of our estimates.

Household composition is introduced into the model [A] by replacing income by income per head and by including as additional explanatory variables the proportion of household members falling in each of nine categories, as follows[4];

- children aged 0 to 4 years

- children aged 5 to 11 years

- males aged 12 to 17 years

- females aged 12 to 17 years

- males aged 18 to 34 years

- males aged 35 to 64 years

- males aged 65 or more years

- females aged 18 to 59 year

- females aged 60 or more years

---

3   These are the heteroskedasticity consistent standard errors described in Eicker [9,10] and White [11]. In the large sample used here they can be employed in a standard asymptotic normal theory based inference without the risk of incurring large errors.

4   These categories are groupings of the categories for which the DHSS define 'Recommended Daily Amounts' of energy intake. In the next section a less coarse grouping is employed.

Also included in the model is the logarithm of the number of persons in the household so that in fact the use of per capita income does not restrict the way in which income enters the model. The resulting model, which is the model used by Deaton [12] and is similar to that used in Chesher and Rees [13], can be expressed as follows;

$$S_i = \frac{e_i}{x} = (\alpha_{i1} n_1 + \alpha_{i2} n_2 + \ldots + \alpha_{i9} n_9) \frac{1}{n} + \beta_i \log\left(\frac{x}{n}\right)$$

$$+ \gamma_i \log(n) + \varepsilon_i \qquad [B]$$

where:

n_r denotes the number of people of type r, r = 1 ... 9

$n = n_1 + n_2 + \ldots + n_9$ represents the total number of household members.

To obtain the results reported here, data for 1988 and 1989 have been pooled. Households reporting net income less than £40 per week were excluded. The resulting sample contained records from 9,089 households. Estimated income coefficients (β_i above) and associated standard errors for nine groups of foods are shown in Table 6.3. A range of foods and food groups has been chosen. As well as 'all food', four broad food groups are studied: 'all meat', 'all fish', 'all vegetables' and 'all fruit'. 'Fresh green vegetables', 'potato products', 'wholemeal bread' and 'white bread' are included to show what happens when narrower food groupings are studied and to provide some cases in which there might be expected to be interesting household composition effects.

It should be noted that the income coefficients are indeed accurately estimated despite the evident scatter in the raw data. All the income coefficients in Table 6.3 are negative indicating that as income rises the proportion of income spent on food falls. At low income levels the model implies that expenditure rises as income rises but at sufficiently high income levels (which vary from one food to another and from one household type to another) expenditure falls with further increases in income. Two reasons for this are diversification in diet and increased incidence of eating out among higher income households.

In the models [A] and [B] the income elasticity of household expenditure on food group i is equal to $1 + \beta_i/S_i$ which depends on the food share, S_i. This elasticity shows the approximate proportionate change in food expenditure that occurs per 1 per cent increase in household income. These elasticities are presented in Table 6.3, calculated at the Survey 1988-89 average food shares. Since the income coefficients are uniformly negative each of the elasticities is less than one. 'All fruit' has the highest income elasticity and is closest to being a 'luxury' among the foods considered here. The income elasticities for 'potato products' and 'white bread' are negative. For the average NFS household these are 'inferior' foods - higher income households tend to spend less on them.

	Estimated income coefficient[a]	Average food shares	Estimated income elasticity[a]
All food	- 0.1565 (0.00266)	0.199	0.21 (0.013)
All meat	- 0.0467 (0.00128)	0.056	0.16 (0.023)
All fish	- 0.0078 (0.00036)	0.011	0.29 (0.032)
All vegetables	- 0.0214 (0.00053)	0.027	0.19 (0.020)
Fresh green veg.	- 0.0022 (0.00013)	0.003	0.36 (0.038)
Potato products	- 0.0027 (0.00013)	0.002	- 0.13 (0.053)
All fruit	- 0.0046 (0.00040)	0.014	0.66 (0.029)
Wholemeal bread	- 0.0011 (0.00011)	0.002	0.37 (0.062)
White bread	- 0.0078 (0.00021)	0.006	- 0.39 (0.037)

Table 6.3 Estimated income coefficients, food shares and income elasticities

(a) Figures in brackets are standard errors

The coefficients on the household size and composition measures are generally quite accurately estimated. The individual coefficients are not reported here because they are not easy to interpret without carrying out further calculations. The effect on food expenditures of adding to the number of household members is quite complex and there are offsetting factors to consider.

We are particularly interested in the effect of household composition while controlling for household income. As household size increases with income held fixed, there are extra mouths to feed and so a tendency for expenditure on foods to increase. But the 'extra mouths' make other demands on the fixed household budget and so there is an offsetting effect pushing food expenditure down. Which of these forces dominates is an empirical matter, depending on the nature of the food under consideration and the size and composition of the household. The NFS data allow us to determine the direction in which food expenditures move as household composition alters for a wide variety of foods.

Tables 6.4 and 6.5 show illustrative calculations based on the estimates of model [B] using the 1988-89 data. The tables show the estimated average effect on food expenditures of adding a single household member to a household. The nine types of household member identified above are considered in turn. Table 6.4 considers a small household, initially containing two persons, an adult male aged 18 to 34 years and an adult female aged 18 to 59 years. Table 6.5 considers a large household, initially containing five members, two adults as in Table 6.5 and also three children of varying ages.

Table 6.4 Estimated changes in expenditures on foods as a member is added to a two person household

percentage of household net income

member type:	child	child	male	female	male	male	male	female	female
aged:	0-4	5-11	12-17	12-17	18-34	35-64	65+	18-59	60+
All food	2.71	3.42	4.51	3.75	4.36	5.95	5.21	5.48	5.42
	(0.289)	(0.249)	(0.383)	(0.360)	(0.189)	(0.227)	(0.221)	(0.182)	(0.210)
All meat	0.36	0.62	0.94	0.65	1.62	2.10	1.84	1.73	1.56
	(0.148)	(0.121)	(0.155)	(0.155)	(0.091)	(0.114)	(0.111)	(0.096)	(0.105)
All fish	0.01	-0.02	0.06	0.04	0.18	0.36	0.36	0.29	0.42
	(0.036)	(0.028)	(0.045)	(0.043)	(0.03)	(0.035)	(0.038)	(0.026)	(0.034)
All veg	0.33	0.53	0.63	0.65	0.54	0.60	0.28	0.67	0.38
	(0.057)	(0.050)	(0.075)	(0.072)	(0.039)	(0.046)	(0.044)	(0.038)	(0.043)
Fresh green veg.	-0.03	0.01	0.03	0.04	0.04	0.10	0.08	0.13	0.16
	(0.011)	(0.010)	(0.015)	(0.016)	(0.010)	(0.012)	(0.013)	(0.009)	(0.010)
Potato products	0.09	0.11	0.13	0.08	0.08	0.06	0.00	0.03	-0.02
	(0.016)	(0.015)	(0.022)	(0.019)	(0.009)	(0.011)	(0.011)	(0.009)	(0.010)
All fruit	0.18	0.26	0.21	0.20	-0.01	0.14	0.27	0.28	0.43
	(0.041)	(0.035)	(0.062)	(0.052)	(0.031)	(0.035)	(0.038)	(0.027)	(0.035)
Wholemeal bread	0.00	0.00	0.02	0.02	0.02	0.04	0.05	0.03	0.05
	(0.010)	(0.009)	(0.015)	(0.015)	(0.008)	(0.010)	(0.012)	(0.010)	(0.011)
White bread	0.10	0.14	0.31	0.21	0.29	0.33	0.26	0.22	0.15
	(0.021)	(0.018)	(0.038)	(0.028)	(0.014)	(0.017)	(0.017)	(0.013)	(0.016)

Figures in brackets are standard errors[5]

Tables 6.4 and 6.5 show the change in expenditure on adding a single household member expressed as a percentage of household income. This is conveniently independent of income and food expenditure. For food i and household member type r it is given by the following expression.

$$\Delta S_i = -\frac{1}{n(n+1)} (\alpha_{i1} n_1 + \alpha_{i2} n_2 + ... + \alpha_{i9} n_9) +$$

$$\frac{\alpha_{ir}}{n+1} - (\beta_i - \gamma_i) \log (1 + \frac{1}{n})$$

5   These are simple to compute because the estimated changes, Δs_i, are linear functions of the estimated coefficients. Heteroskedasticity robust variance estimates are used here too.

Table 6.5 Estimated changes in expenditure on foods as a member is added to a five person household

percentage of household net income

member type:	child	child	male	female	male	male	male	female	female
aged:	0-4	5-11	12-17	12-17	18-34	35-64	65+	18-59	60+
All food	1.52	1.87	2.42	2.04	2.35	3.14	2.77	2.91	2.88
	(0.121)	(0.114)	(0.160)	(0.190)	(0.148)	(0.156)	(0.146)	(0.145)	(0.147)
All meat	0.41	0.54	0.70	0.55	1.04	1.27	1.15	1.09	1.01
	(0.060)	(0.053)	(0.064)	(0.079)	(0.075)	(0.080)	(0.072)	(0.077)	(0.075)
All fish	0.06	0.04	0.09	0.07	0.14	0.23	0.24	0.20	0.27
	(0.015)	(0.013)	(0.018)	(0.023)	(0.022)	(0.024)	(0.024)	(0.021)	(0.023)
All veg	0.17	0.27	0.32	0.33	0.27	0.30	0.14	0.34	0.19
	(0.023)	(0.023)	(0.031)	(0.037)	(0.030)	(0.031)	(0.029)	(0.029)	(0.030)
Fresh green veg.	0.01	0.02	0.03	0.04	0.04	0.07	0.06	0.08	0.10
	(0.005)	(0.004)	(0.006)	(0.008)	(0.008)	(0.008)	(0.008)	(0.007)	(0.008)
Potato products	0.03	0.04	0.05	0.02	0.02	0.01	-0.02	0.00	-0.03
	(0.007)	(0.007)	(0.009)	(0.010)	(0.008)	(0.007)	(0.007)	(0.007)	(0.008)
All fruit	0.06	0.10	0.07	0.07	-0.04	0.04	0.10	0.11	0.19
	(0.018)	(0.016)	(0.026)	(0.028)	(0.022)	(0.023)	(0.024)	(0.021)	(0.022)
Wholemeal bread	0.00	0.01	0.01	0.01	0.01	0.02	0.03	0.02	0.03
	(0.004)	(0.004)	(0.006)	(0.008)	(0.006)	(0.007)	(0.007)	(0.007)	(0.007)
White bread	0.06	0.08	0.16	0.11	0.15	0.17	0.14	0.11	0.08
	(0.009)	(0.009)	(0.015)	(0.015)	(0.011)	(0.012)	(0.012)	(0.011)	(0.012)

Figures in brackets are standard errors[5]

The figures in Tables 6.4 and 6.5 are summarised in the bar charts of Figure 6.6.

Figure 6.6
Extra percentage of
income spent on food
as one person of the
indicated type is added
to a family

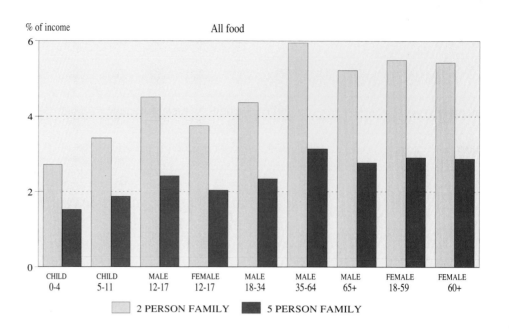

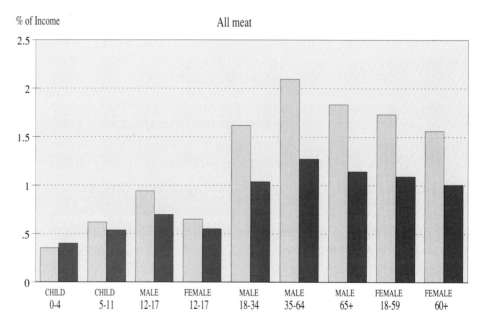

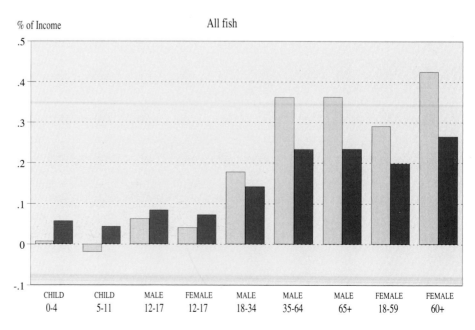

Figure 6.6 continued

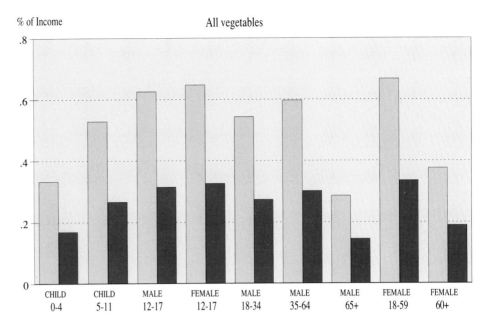

% of Income — All vegetables

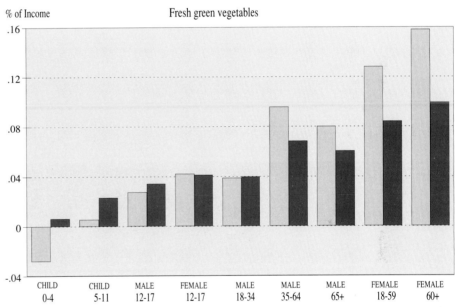

% of Income — Fresh green vegetables

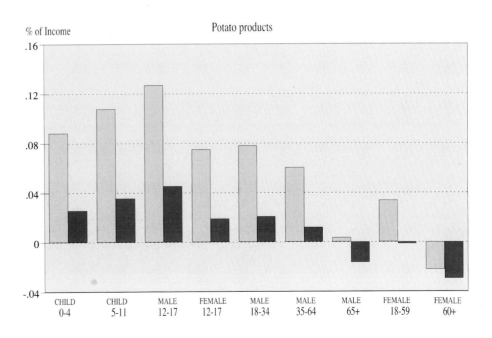

% of Income — Potato products

Figure 6.6 continued

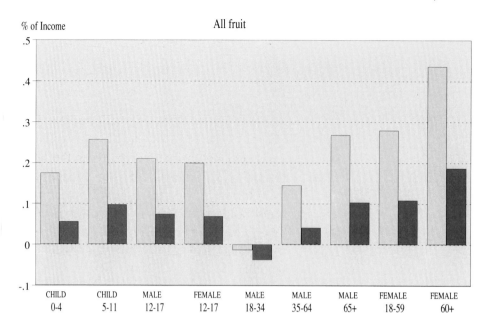

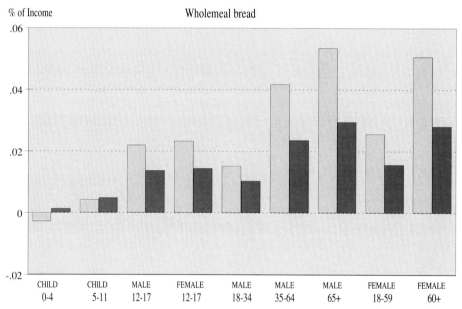

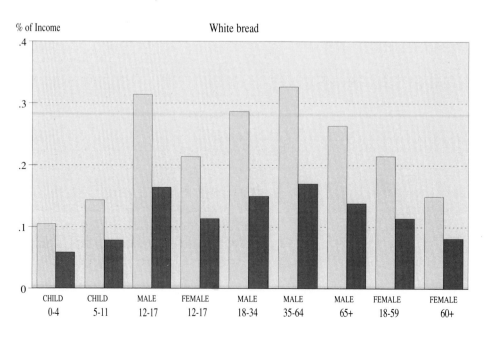

A number of points should be noted. First, observe that in most cases the addition of a household member does lead to an increase in food expenditure. The 'hungry mouths' dominate the other demands on the household budget. However the increase is uniformly smaller when the household is already a large one. This may be in part due to economies of scale in the provision of food for consumption in the household, but it is surely also due to economising on food expenditure as the extra household member burdens the household budget with demands for clothes and space and other goods as well as food. These figures should not be taken to suggest that larger households eat less than smaller households with the same income, or even less well, just that they eat 'less expensively'. The next section examines whether the quantity of food (measured by calories of energy consumed) is reduced as income is reduced.

Of course, the percentages by which expenditure alters vary greatly as we go from broad food groups to narrowly defined foods. An extra household member causes expenditure on 'all food' to rise by between 3 per cent and 6 per cent in small families and by slightly more than half this in large families. For a minor item in the food budget like 'wholemeal bread' the changes are much smaller. However, in many cases the changes are accurately estimated as the standard errors in Tables 6.4 and 6.5 show.

The effect of adding a household member depends on the type of member involved. For 'all food' the impact of a household member increases with age. For adolescents it is higher for boys than for girls but among adults, gender related differences are small. Note that these figures refer to expenditure on food brought into the home and that the incidence of eating out may be age and gender related.

For specific foods and food groups there are quite noticeable age differences. For example, the impact on meat expenditure is much smaller when a child is added to a household than when an adult is added. The difference is even more marked for 'all fish' - many parents will recognise this phenomenon. Green vegetables and wholemeal bread follow a similar pattern - these do not seem to be favourites with British children in 1988-89, but for potato products the effect is in the opposite direction. Again many couples will have noticed that their kitchen has more chips and crisps once they become parents.

It is encouraging to see that the NFS data can reveal these plausible differences. More importantly the NFS also allows the measurement of the magnitude of these effects and the tracking of them through time as well as observation of the way tastes for food change as one generation succeeds another and as peoples' attitudes to foods change. In the example in the next section the problem of detecting change in behaviour is of central importance.

Household composition and diet

As more and more studies suggest links between diet and health there is increasing interest in the nutritional components of individuals' diets and in the ways in which these change through time. Even though the NFS does not record consumption of foods or nutrients by individuals, the household food acquisition data it obtains can be used to estimate intakes of nutrients by household members of different types. This is demonstrated in this section by drawing on results reported in [3].

The key to this analysis is the observation that; (a) on average households' rates of consumption of nutrients from household supplies are equal to rates at which nutrients enter the household food supplies; and (b) to a first approximation, the average rate of household consumption of a nutrient is equal to the sum of the average rates of consumption by each of the household's members. This allows the amount of a nutrient acquired by a NFS household in a survey week, A_H say, to be expressed as:

$$A_H = \delta_0 + \delta_1 n_1 + \delta_2 n_2 + ... + \delta_r n_r + \varepsilon \qquad [C]$$

where:
A_H is the amount of a nutrient acquired by household H
n_r denotes the number of household members of type r, r = 1 ... 9.

The coefficient δ_i can be interpreted as the average rate of consumption of the nutrient per household member of type i. The constant term, δ_0, can be interpreted as the rate of consumption by visitors and by pets. As in the last section, ε is a random disturbance capturing variation across households in long run average rates of consumption and also variation within households around these long run average rates of consumption across time.

The coefficients of the model [C] (i.e. household member type specific rates of nutrient intake) can be estimated by regression analysis using data on amounts of nutrients in the recorded household food supplies and information on household composition. The nutrient information is obtained by applying regularly updated nutrient conversion factors to the quantities of foods of different types that NFS households record in their diaries. The estimation procedure, the interpretation of the model and extensions to it are described in [3] and they are summarised in the 1989 report of the NFS Committee [1]. Here just a few illustrative results will be presented.

Figures 6.9, 6.10 and 6.11 show respectively estimated intakes of energy and estimated rates of consumption of fats and of polyunsaturated fatty acids for 25 types of household member classified by age, gender and activity status. The estimates relate to 1979-80 and 1988-89 so that rates of consumption can be compared across the decade as well as across household member types. These graphs have some striking features.

68

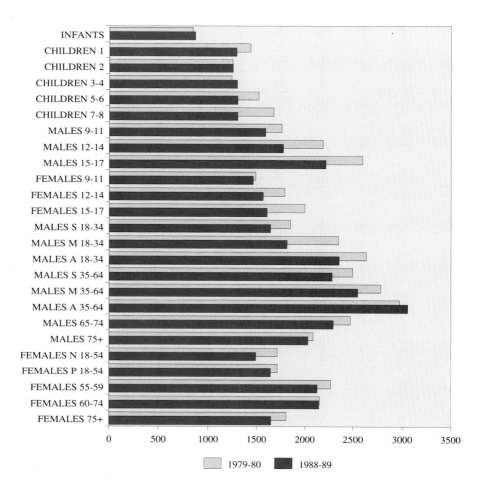

Figure 6.7
Daily energy consumption
(kcal/person/day)

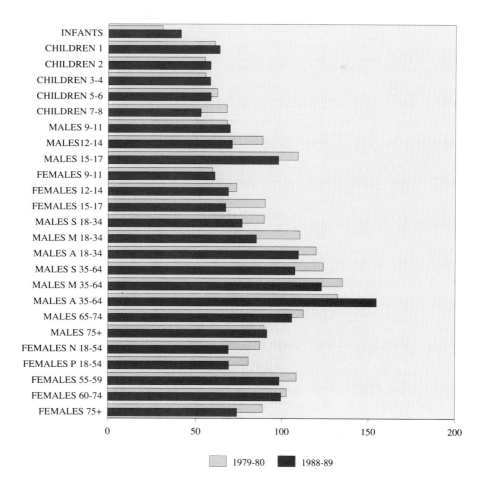

Figure 6.8
Daily fat consumption
(g/person/day)

Figure 6.9
Daily consumption of
polyunsaturated fatty acids
(g/person/day)

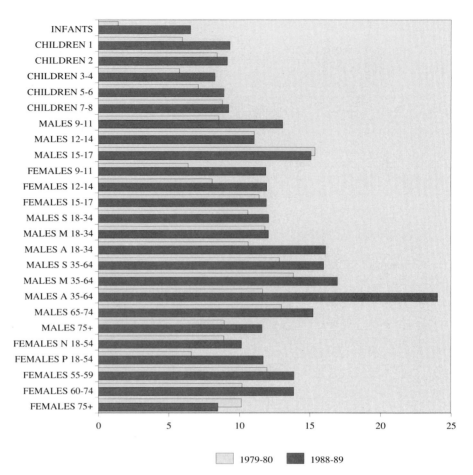

First, the rates of consumption of energy and fats increase with age and with the strenuousness of individuals' activities (S is sedentary, M is moderately active and A is active occupations). Among adults, they are higher for males than for females. They show very similar variation to that found in the DHSS 'Recommended Daily Amounts'. It is clear that both energy intakes and fat consumption have declined during the 1980s, but more so for some types of household member than for others. For example, reductions have been greater for adults than for children.

Second, the substantial increase in the rate of consumption of poly-unsaturated fatty acids should be noted. This is probably the major dietary change of the decade and one which is in line with the Committee on the Medical Aspects of Food Policy recommendation [14] to increase the ratio of polyunsaturated fatty acids to saturated fatty acids. Again the NFS data reveal that some groups have been affected more than others.

The NFS is believed to be the longest running continuous food survey in the world and its continuity is one of its most important attributes. This is demonstrated by the final graphs in this paper which show time series of estimated dietary indicators obtained by estimating the model [C] for each year from 1979 to 1989.

Figures 6.12 and 6.13 present the estimated time paths of six indicators for respectively, non-pregnant females aged 18 to 54 years and moderately active males aged 18 to 34 years. Linear trends have been fitted to each sequence of indicators and drawn with solid rather than dotted lines where they are statistically significantly increasing or decreasing. Frequently the trends are significant even though year on year changes are small; a particularly striking point is the relatively tight variation in the estimates around steady trends.

Figure 6.10 Time paths for dietary indicators: Females not pregnant aged 18-54 years

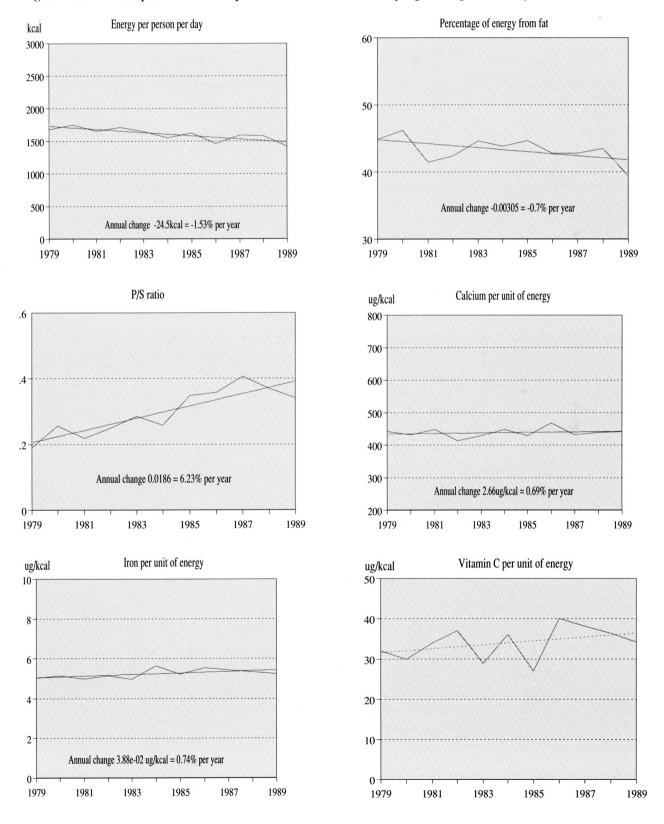

For females there is a clear steady decline in energy intake and in the proportion of energy derived from fat. However at over 0.4 this is still well above the Department of Health recommended level of 0.35. Females also show a slight increase in iron consumption per unit of energy and a marked rise in the P/S ratio, the ratio of the amounts of polyunsaturated to saturated fatty acids. For the males considered here (the results do vary across subgroups of males), energy intakes have fallen quite substantially but the proportion of energy obtained from fat has actually risen during the 1980s. As for women, the P/S ratio has increased markedly and there are signs of a very slight increase in iron and calcium per unit of energy.

Figure 6.11 Time paths for dietary indicators: Moderately active males aged 18-34 years

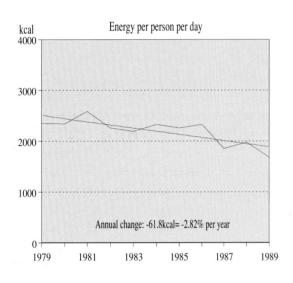

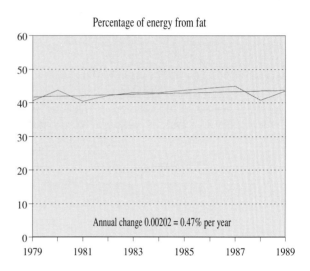

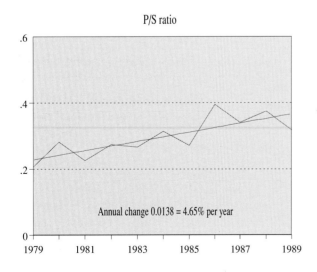

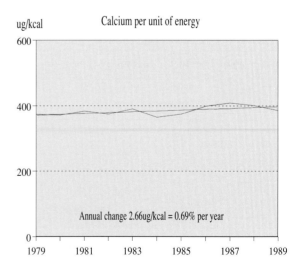

Figure 6.11 continued

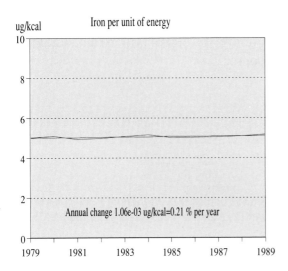

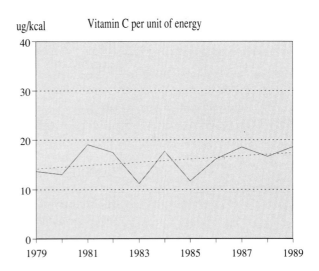

Finally model [C] can be extended to include terms for income. When this is done, very small income coefficients are estimated and, for most nutrients (vitamin C is an exception), they indicate that nutrient intakes *fall* very slightly as income increases. This perverse result almost certainly arises because the NFS data refer to nutrients in household supplies of food. Higher income households probably get more nutrients outside the home than others, first because 'social' eating out is a luxury and second because eating out associated with employment will increase with the number of earners in a household and so with household income. When the data are converted for the number of meals taken from non-household food supplies, the income effects disappear except for vitamin C which does seem to be consumed at a higher rate in high income households. It was noted in the previous section that fruit was, relative to many other foods, a luxury in the economic sense, so this result is to be expected.

Concluding remarks

The National Food Survey represents a unique source of knowledge concerning the food purchasing behaviour of British households. It covers a wide range of households and when subjected to careful analysis it can be seen to contain a wealth of information concerning the relationship between household size and composition and food expenditure as well as nutrient intakes and related dietary indicators.

The continuity of the Survey and the breadth of topics it covers allows researchers from many disciplines to study the dynamics of consumer behaviour, trends and changes in tastes, and changes in consumers' awareness of diet and its components.

In this paper the ability of the NFS data to reveal the impact of income and household composition on food expenditure has been demonstrated and it has been shown that the NFS data can give information about average rates of consumption of nutrients for people of different ages and gender.

It has been the intention of this paper to demonstrate the utility of the NFS in the hope that, by doing so, others will be encouraged to exploit this most valuable resource.

REFERENCES

[1] Ministry of Agriculture, Fisheries and Food (1990), *Household Food Consumption and Expenditure, 1989,* annual report of the National Food Survey Committee, HMSO.

[2] Ministry of Food (1952), *Domestic Food Consumption and Expenditure, 1950,* annual report of the National Food Survey Committee, HMSO.

[3] Chesher, A D (1990), *Nutrients in British Household Food Supplies: Variation Across Households and Changes During the 1980s,* unpublished report prepared for the Ministry of Agriculture, Fisheries and Food.

[4] Cleveland, W S (1979), *Robust Locally Weighted Regression and Smoothing Scatter Plots,* Journal of the American Statistical Association, 74, 829-836.

[5] Becker, R A, Chambers, J M and Wilks, A R (1988), *The New S Lanaguage,* Wadsworth & Brooks/Cole, Pacific Grove, California.

[6] Working, H (1943), *Statistical Laws of Family Expenditure,* Journal of the American Statistical Association, 38, 43-56.

[7] Leser, C V (1963), *Forms of Engel Functions,* Econometrica, 31, 694-703.

[8] Deaton, A S and Muellbauer, J (1980), *An Almost Ideal Demand System,* American Economic Review, 70, 312-326.

[9] Eicker, F (1963), *Asymptotic Normality and Consistency of the Least Squares Estimators for Families of Linear Regressions,* Annals of Mathematical Statistics, 34, 447-456.

[10] Eicker, F (1967), *Limit Theorems for Regressions with Unequal and Dependent Errors,* Proceedings of the Fourth Berkeley Symposium on Mathematical Statistics and Probability, Vol. 1, Berkeley: University of California.

[11] White, H (1980), *A Heteroskedasticity-consistent Covariance Matrix Estimator and a Direct Test for Heteroskedasticity of Unknown Form,* Econometrica, 48, 817-838.

[12] Deaton, A S (1988), *The Allocation of Goods Within the Household,* Living Standards Measurement, Working Paper No. 39, The World Bank, Washington D.C.

[13] Chesher, A D and Rees, H J B (1987), *Income Elasticities of Demands for Food in Great Britain,* Journal of Agricultural Economics, 38, 435-448.

[14] Department of Health and Social Security (1984), *Diet and Cardiovascular Disease,* HMSO.

The Value
of the
National Food Survey

CHAPTER 7

An Economist's View

John Slater

Introduction

In considering the value of the National Food Survey (NFS), there are a number of general points which need to be made. The first is that the NFS is designed to provide information for government and the data are used by government for a wide variety of purposes. However, the information collected is also of value to those outside government. It is made available through published reports, for academic research through the ESRC data archive and on a commercial basis.

Clearly, those who are responsible for advising Ministers need information which is as accurate and reliable as possible and some aspects of the process of trying to ensure accurate data are considered in the next section. However, the NFS is one of three major household surveys conducted by government, the others being the Family Expenditure Survey (FES) [1] and the General Household Survey (GHS) [2]: it benefits from the expertise derived from these and other major government surveys. In particular, the NFS benefits from the professionalism of the Office of Population Censuses and Surveys (OPCS) and the commercial companies which undertake the fieldwork for the survey.

The second point is that advisers in government try to avoid relying on only one source of information. No survey can be 100 per cent accurate but we can have more confidence if the results are broadly consistent with other data either collected by government or by others outside the industry. For instance, we are able to cross check NFS data against less detailed data on expenditure on food from the FES. As Figure 7.1 demonstrates, the fit is remarkably close. The lack of precise comparability on levels reflects the difficulty of ensuring common definitions in the treatment of the grey area of food which may, or may not, be consumed away from the home.

£ per person per week

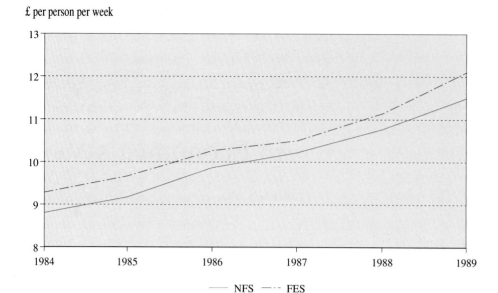

Movements in household consumption can also be cross checked against other information, such as supplies available for consumption as measured by balance sheet data. A comparison for sheepmeat is given in Figure 7.2 and demonstrates a remarkably close fit. In practice such a precise match would not be expected because of differences in timing and coverage. Added to which, if products are sold in more processed form, the volume change is likely to be smaller for the household consumption data over the longer term. However, there can be more confidence in the data series if seasonal movements and turning points are similar and if trends move broadly in line over the medium term.

Figure 7.2
Comparison of NFS and
balance sheet data for
sheepmeat purchases:
United Kingdom

Index 1985 Q1=100

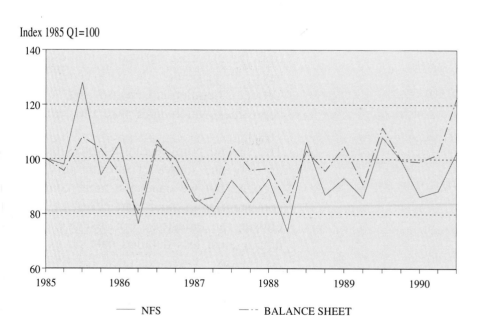

In other words, while the NFS is used for many purposes, it is rarely the only source for any one purpose.

A third point which is particularly relevant to data used by economists and statisticians in government is that it should be, as far as possible, representative of the population as a whole and as complete as possible in its coverage; for most purposes, government needs aggregate and comprehensive information. That is why the government's large household surveys are based, almost without exception, on random samples rather than household panels. However, this does mean that standard errors are likely to be larger than with panel survey estimates and greater care has to be taken in interpreting short term movements, especially if the data are disaggregated.

Main uses of NFS data by government

There are three main areas of use to which NFS data are put by economists and statisticians in government; the construction of economic indicators; the monitoring and assessment of trends and the analysis of policy options. These are each considered in turn.

Construction of Economic Indicators

The NFS is an important source of data for the construction of economic indicators.

(a) Consumers expenditure: Data from the NFS are aggregated for the main food groups to provide estimates of consumers' expenditure on food at both current and constant prices. These data are supplemented by information on foods not included in the survey, currently confectionery and soft drinks. The aggregate estimates of household expenditure on food are inputs into the construction of one of the government's main economic indicators of growth, Gross Domestic Product by the expenditure method, GDP(E).

The current price estimates are derived from 'raw' NFS data on expenditure, expressed on a 'per head per week' basis, and using year specific grossing up factors. The latter are obtained by adjusting annual estimates of the resident population within the UK to exclude, for instance, foreign visitors, persons staying in community establishments, such as boarding schools, hospitals or prisons, and UK residents temporarily overseas. The constant price estimates are obtained by multiplying the recorded volume of purchases of each good by its price in a given base year.

(b) The Retail Prices Index: Data from the NFS are also used in the construction of a second major economic indicator, the Retail Prices Index (RPI). The RPI is constructed by weighting together prices of a representative basket of good and services purchased by the 'typical' household. NFS data are used in both the determination of the weights for the index and in the selection of appropriate indicators.

The weights for most items, including those for the main food groups, are derived from FES data. Information from the NFS is, however, used to derive sub sector weights for food items. This is particularly important for fruit and vegetables where variable monthly weights are applied. For example, when the home tomato crop is at its peak in June, tomatoes have a weight of 2.5 within the RPI. As domestic supplies fall off this weight is reduced so that by September it has dropped to 1.8. Although the weights attached to individual items change seasonally, the total weight for the food group remains the same during the year since seasonal variations in the purchase of any one item tend to be compensated for by offsetting purchases of similar items.

Analyses of NFS data are also used to decide which foods should be selected as indicator items. Food tends to have a proportionately high number of indicators reflecting the large number of relatively low priced items and the variability of price movements between items. While some basic foods have remained as indicators for many years, the dramatic changes in the foods available for consumption necessitate a continual process of updating. For some groups, the number of indicators can be reduced but, for others, additional indicators are needed as illustrated in Table 7.3. In particular, following the report of the Retail Prices Index Advisory Committee in 1986 [3], steps were taken to extend the range of fresh fruit and vegetables whose prices were included in the index. Previously, foods which were not available for the whole of the year were excluded. Analysis of NFS data led to the selection of lettuce, avocado pears, grapes, nectarines and kiwi fruit as new indicators and enabled appropriate weights to be calculated for these items.

Table 7.3
Indicator items in the
Retail Prices Index

		1980	1990
FRUIT		Apples, cooking	Apples, cooking
		Apples, dessert	Apples, dessert
		Pears	Pears
		Oranges	Oranges
			Strawberries
			Plums
			Grapes
			Nectarines
			Avocado pears
			Kiwi fruit
PRESERVES		Marmalade	Marmalade
		Strawberry jam	Strawberry jam
		Raspberry jam	Honey
		Plum jam	
		Blackcurrant jam	
		Golden Syrup	

(c) Other government series: NFS data contribute to many other statistical series on a regular or less frequent basis. For instance, the quantity data available from the NFS allow constant price series to be calculated directly for some parts of the Index of Production.

Monitoring and
assessment of trends

The NFS represents a long standing and comprehensive database of household food consumption and expenditure and is used extensively for monitoring and assessing trends. Given its continuity over a long period, the NFS provides a relatively quick means of identifying and quantifying changes in consumption patterns - both those which may be regarded as evolutionary, such as the shift away from whole milk towards low fat milks, and those which occur as a result of sudden shocks to the system such as health scares - real or imagined. It effectively provides an invaluable source of information on consumers' behaviour with respect to food.

Associated with this monitoring process is the preparation of short and medium terms forecasts. As well as forecasts made for internal purposes, the Department is often called upon to supply forecasts of consumption to international bodies such as OECD. The NFS furnishes quantitative data of household consumption which, when grossed up, provides a base from which to forecast. An illustration of forecasts for UK meat consumption is given in Figure 7.4.

Figure 7.4
Forecasts of the
consumption of meat
in the United Kingdom

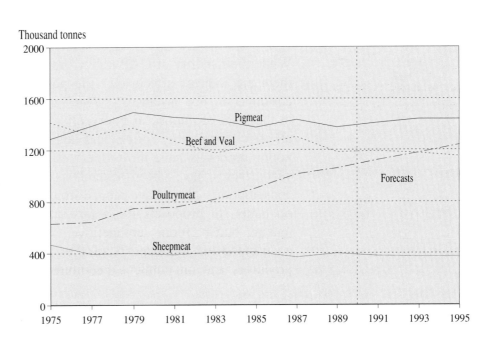

The Survey data also provide the basis for estimating elasticities - own price, cross price and income - and residual underlying trends which can be used in constructing such forecasts. This type of work has already been considered in earlier sections.

Analysis of
policy options

Much of the work of economists within the Ministry is concerned with assessing the likely effects of policy proposals which emanate from Brussels, other member states or from the government's own initiatives and some of the general policy areas are set out in Figure 7.5. The NFS provides an ideal base from which to judge the possible effects of such proposals on consumption and consumers.

Figure 7.5
Types of policy options
assessed

---

1. Policy options aimed primarily at farm output / income

    (a) Support prices

    (b) Quotas and set aside

    (c) Green pound devaluations

2. Policy options aimed primarily at consumption

    (a) Consumer subsidies

    (b) Welfare schemes

    (c) Import taxes

    (d) Manufacturer subsidies

While the majority of CAP policy proposals are aimed at the producer, there are indirect effects on the population both as taxpayers and consumers. For instance, changes in the level of the green pound, in the level of quotas, in intervention arrangements or export refunds, all affect commodity prices and households' demand for food. Other policy proposals have more direct effects on the consumer. In recent years, there have been several proposals aimed more directly at consumption. These have ranged from consumer subsidies, for instance on butter, to proposals for a fats tax with the primary objective of making butter more competitive with margarine. NFS data have contributed to assessments of the likely impact on consumers, on producers and on public expenditure.

By way of illustration the use of a tax on a product to stimulate the consumption of a substitute depends for its efficiency on a high cross price elasticity. Otherwise, a disproportionately high tax would be required to achieve a significant impact on demand for the substitute, implying substantial market distortions. In the case of butter and margarine, the NFS data have for some years indicated cross price elasticities which are very low. This has been supported by other more recent studies. As the UK government has long argued, an oils and fats tax designed to raise the price of margarine would be an extremely inefficient way of reducing the EC butter surplus.

Conclusions

It has not been possible to do more than indicate in very general terms how economists and statisticians use the NFS data. The construction of economic indicators represents an extremely important use. The indicators in question - consumers' expenditure, retail prices and the index of production - are central to macro-economic policy. The data provide an important tool in monitoring and assessing food consumption trends and in evaluating policy alternatives. The latter is inevitably more ad-hoc. However, in the absence of the NFS data, it would be extremely difficult to provide assessments of the kind frequently needed by policy makers in evaluating developments and in assessing the options that are open to them.

REFERENCES

[1] Central Statistical Office (1990), *Family Expenditure Survey 1989*, HMSO.

[2] Office of Population, Censuses and Surveys (1990), *General Household Survey 1988*, HMSO.

[3] Department of Employment (1986), *Methodological Issues Affecting the Retail Price Index*, Report of Retail Prices Advisory Committee, HMSO.

CHAPTER 8

A Health Scientist's View

Martin Wiseman and Robert Wenlock

Introduction

This view of the value of the National Food Survey (NFS) is given from the perspective of a particular kind of health scientist, that is one from the Department of Health. There are many other kinds of health scientists, each of which may well make different uses of the huge amount of data generated by the NFS.

The Department of Health role

To understand the value of the NFS to the Department of Health, it is important to understand the context in which the information it generates is used. As far as nutrition is concerned, the Department of Health's role is three-fold:

- to ensure that government has an adequate understanding of the relationship between diet, nutrition and health

- to ensure, via surveillance and appraisal of the results of surveillance, that government understands the population's nutritional status

- to develop policy and programmes to reduce diet-related diseases and disabilities. It is apparent that, in this area, surveillance provides the linchpin for policy making.

Monitoring nutrition

Nutrition is an area that crosses many boundaries both in science and government. Nutritional health depends not only on the food consumed but also on the consumer's particular response to it. In order to understand the relationships between diets and health (and disease), we must know not only about the individual's physiology, but also about food consumption and the composition of that food. In the latter two areas, the Ministry of Agriculture, Fisheries and Food (MAFF) plays an important role and, in the area of the food consumption, the NFS is pre-eminent. Data from the NFS provide regular, up to date and accurate information on average food purchases by the population. It is known from comparison of the NFS results with those from formal dietary surveys that, in general, nutrients available from households' acquisitions of food reflects accurately the nutrient intakes by the population.

The NFS is especially useful because it provides data on the trends in intakes of both foods and nutrients, not only in the short term but also over the longer term - and now up to 50 years ago. This is a key component in the examination of the relationships between diet and disease within the population. One of the particular values of the NFS is that it provides very robust data, which can be analysed in relation to a number of other parameters, such as region and income. Again long term trends can be demonstrated. For some time, it has been known that there are differences in the incidence of certain diseases, such as cardiovascular disease, across the country (more in Scotland and the North, less in London and the South East) [1]. The NFS has shown only small differences in nutrient intake (in spite of greater differences in dietary patterns) between these areas. This suggests that differences in disease mortality may be due to factors other than the conventional dietary risk factors. This is a useful pointer for further research.

Knowledge of these trends is used not only to identify areas of potential concern but also to monitor the effects of policies. It has been used as a tool for many of the reports emanating from the Committee on Medical Aspects of Food Policy (COMA). Even as long ago as 1968 its predecessor committee, the Committee on Medical and Nutritional Aspects of Food Policy, used information from the NFS in its report on *A Pilot Survey of the Nutrition of Young Children in 1963* [2]. The COMA sub-committee on nutritional surveillance found data from the NFS essential to all three of its reports published in 1973, 1981 and 1988 [3,4,5]. The more recent COMA reports on specific aspects of diet and health, particularly the report on *Diet and Cardiovascular Disease* in 1984 [6], used data on trends in energy, proteins, fat, carbohydrate, fatty acids and dietary fibre consumption from the NFS in coming to its conclusions [7]. The COMA report on *Dietary Sugars in Human Disease* also used the NFS to show trends in packet sugar purchases since 1940 and the contribution of food groups to intakes of individual sugars [7]. Currently the results from the NFS are providing one of the most important sets of information on which the deliberations of the current COMA Panel on Recommended Daily Amounts for Food Energy and Nutrients are based.

Without doubt our understanding of diet's role in the health of the population depends to a greater or lesser extent on our knowledge of current dietary trends. The National Food Survey is one of our best tools for that purpose.

REFERENCES

[1] Department of Health (1990), *On the State of the Public Health for the Year 1989*, London, HMSO.

[2] Ministry of Health (1968), *A Pilot Study of the Nutrition of Young Children in 1963*, HMSO.

[3] Department of Health and Social Security (1973), *First Report by the Sub-Committee on Nutritional Surveillance*, HMSO.

[4] Department of Health and Social Security (1981), *Second Report of the Sub-Committee on Nutritional Surveillance*, HMSO.

[5] Department of Health (1988), *Third Report of the Sub-Committee on Nutritional Surveillance*, HMSO.

[6] Department of Health and Social Security (1984), *Diet and Cardiovascular Disease*, HMSO.

[7] Department of Health (1989), *Dietary Sugars and Human Disease*, HMSO.

CHAPTER 9

A View from the Food Industry

Ivor Hunt

Introduction

It is a privilege to be asked to contribute to the 50th birthday celebrations of the National Food Survey (NFS) and to present the view of someone who has worked in the food industry for many years on how NFS data are used in the commercial sector.

The first thing to say is that the food sector is large and diverse; it makes a significant contribution to GDP and, even excluding catering, accounts for nearly 9 per cent of the labour force. Furthermore, it is estimated that expenditure on food represents around 18 per cent of total consumers' expenditure, of which 12 per cent is on food eaten at home. Simplistically, the sector can be split into three distinct parts; production; processing and manufacturing; and distribution and retailing (Table 9.1). Each is overlaid by a complex network of rules and regulations to ensure that the ultimate consumer enjoys good wholesome food no matter from where it comes.

Table 9.1
Composition of the food and drink sector

	Contribution to GDP[a]	Employment[b]	
		Overall	Within food industry
	per cent	per cent	per cent
Production - mainly agriculture, horticulture and fishing	1.4	2.1	24
Processing - packing, refining and manufacturing	2.5	2.0	23
Distribution - wholesaling and retailing	2.9	4.6	53
Total for sector	6.8	8.7	100

(a) 1988

(b) September 1990

The changing market

But not only is the food industry large and complex, it is also changing rapidly. This is not the place to comment on those changes as they affect farming and food manufacturing or processing except to say that clearly for both, current changes are fundamental. Throughout the timespan, or life, of the NFS (but in no way connected to it as far as I know), farmers have been encouraged through a variety of schemes and subsidies to become more efficient and productive. Because of their vital role in generating one of life's basics, they have operated within a regime in which they have enjoyed protection and support. However, this is a regime which, powerful as it is, now seems to be under more pressure than ever before - as we have seen from the recent GATT talks.

Food processors along with all other manufacturers are also moving towards a brave new world - the new world of 1992. Fifteen or twenty years ago they were resenting the evolution of stronger and more professional food retailers and some, at least, felt threatened. (Although I should add that in my view this is less of a concern now than once it was). Now they have before them a great opportunity with many already working towards genuinely operating on a European scale - unlike retailers who develop and evolve within the culture of a country and can be restricted by that culture. Generally retailers find great difficulty in transferring a successful formula across national boundaries.

So what of the changes as they affect retailing. Of course in respect of a birthday, it is appropriate to try and relate those changes to conception; that is to look back over the 50 years of the NFS. That takes us back to 1940 when food retailing was very different from the present day. Indeed it was even more constrained then by the special regulations in place. At that time, J. Sainsbury had about 250 shops which is not very different from the present number. However, none were self service; this did not arrive until the early '50s. The company stocked less than 1,000 lines and customers queued at marble counters which are still remembered by many today. There were different queues for bacon, butter and so on. Sales were £20 million then; they have increased by no less than 30 times in real terms in the past 50 years.

But more interesting, and certainly more relevant, are the changes that have taken place over the last 10 years. Sainsbury's larger stores, such as the new store at Tunbridge Wells, now stock 14,000 lines including different sizes and flavours - up from 7,000 ten years ago. Typically about 1,000 new lines have been introduced each year in recent years and the number is expected to increase to nearer 2,000 in the coming year. The introductions range from genuinely innovative new products to additional sizes and flavours of existing lines. That there is such a large product development programme, whilst the total range is confined to 14,000 or so, illustrates the rate of change that is taking place. This is an accelerating process and reflects the changing attitudes of all the individuals that go to make up the population. Factors influencing these changes, like increased foreign travel, greater media exposure (especially television) and better education (often hard to believe), are all well documented. The outcome is a restless quest for greater individuality - people want to be different from the Joneses, not to keep up with them. Incidentally it is interesting to see how the motor car industry has dealt with this change. It has preserved the production advantages of mass producing basic models and then offered a wide range of variants; there was a time when it was possible to buy some 50 different types or variant of Ford Escort. The food industry's response has been to widen its range.

The need for information

Where does the NFS fit into all of this? Well, for a large and diverse industry that is changing fast, the need for reliable information is paramount. What sort of information? Well I think there are three broad types:

- an assessment of the economy in which we operate;

- the need to track the markets in which we operate;

- the need to know about the behaviour and attitudes of consumers and our competitors' customers.

The NFS is mainly concerned with the second and third of these although it does not distinguish purchases from different outlets.

For the farming sector, there must be a need to understand long term trends in food consumption and their implications for the future. Farmers need to answer such questions as to whether or not meat consumption has peaked with the greater acceptance and perceived benefits of vegetarian alternatives. For example, a small but steady move towards fish, pulses, quorn, cheese and eggs, etc, is seen. Then there is the general question of relevance to all three sectors of the industry. To what extent are we seeing a trend towards 'less but better' eating - a trend evident in some other markets? To what extent is this true of food markets or will it become true of food markets in the same way that, generally, people are drinking 'less but better' tables wines? You may think that this is a poor example because of the special circumstances that may have accelerated the process for alcoholic drinks but, from my perspective, it is a trend that is beginning to move in many food sectors, eg: Traditional Beef, Tenderlean Lamb, speciality breads, fruit and vegetables, etc. If this is so, then the NFS is an obvious vehicle for monitoring these changes. Any ways in which it can be modified to reveal such changes would be illuminating for *all* sectors of the industry.

The processing and retailing parts of the industry seem to have a never ending - certainly an ever increasing - demand for market knowledge. Information is obtained from a variety of sources, including the NFS. The NFS is important because it is comprehensive, covering all food consumption. Furthermore its *consistency* of coverage and methodology over time are great strengths. Through the NFS one really can monitor long term trends in a way that cannot be achieved through any other survey. And here I would add that I, personally, value the statistical rigour and openness about statistical limitations that I have always associated with the NFS. If I were to mention one concern I do have, it is the extent to which the results from the NFS may be overstated. I know, from experience, that household panels always overstate purchasing when they are set up and that it takes a few weeks for the measure to settle down.

Other sources of information

What are the other sources of market information?

Firstly there is the Family Expenditure Survey where coverage is as wide but the detail on food is less than for the NFS. It has its value to the large general food retailer as a basis for judging performance in some non-food markets such as toiletries and off licence.

Then there's the market data available through market research agencies, the principle ones being the A C Nielson Company and AGB Research. Of course, these are commercial organisations and collect that information which they can readily sell at a profit which does not always lead to consistency over time. This is unlike the NFS where other considerations have ensured the long term stability which, as I have said, is a strength. These commercial measures provide a great deal of information about the branded goods markets but rather less about the more fragmented perishable markets; this is a limitation which they are seeking to overcome in the new services that they are developing and introducing. Both companies operate audits of the sales through retail outlets from which I believe we get the most reliable estimates of the *size* of the defined market being measured and some details, for example brand shares, in those markets. But, because retailers are loathe to have their sales data exposed in such audits, they do *not* reveal information about the performance of individual retail organisations.

Both companies also use household panels to collect market data and these have many features in common with the NFS. Through them the research agencies are able to publish the shares that major retailers achieve within defined markets. However, more significantly, the advantages of a full panel operation, in which the same households remain members continuously, is that it allows analysis over time of the purchasing patterns of individual or groups of households. In the dynamic market that I talked of earlier, this is especially important. For example, brand switching analyses can be undertaken. The characteristics of households which try new products compared to those which are more traditional in their consumption can be identified and assessments made of the extent to which the products are generating repeat purchases. The impact of promotional activity such as store coupons, product demonstrations, media advertising, etc., can be analysed.

I do not believe that the measures of market size are as accurate as those derived from audits but the market insights can be invaluable.

The role of the NFS

The NFS, because of the way it is collected, cannot go into such detailed analyses. Its value for food retailers is in setting the context for judging own trading performance in markets that are not well documented by commercial agencies. Figures 9.2 to 9.4 give you some idea of one of the ways in which we look at the data.

Figure 9.2
Comparison of trends in cheese between Sainsbury and the NFS

1982/1983 = 100

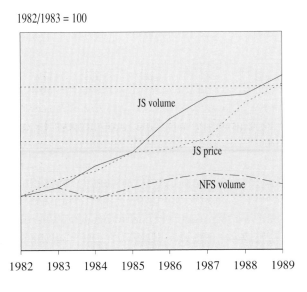

1982   1983   1984   1985   1986   1987   1988   1989

Figure 9.3
Comparison of trends in poultry between Sainsbury and the NFS

1982/1983 = 100

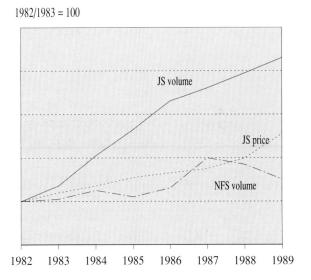

1982   1983   1984   1985   1986   1987   1988   1989

Figure 9.4
Comparison of trends in eggs between Sainsbury and the NFS

1982/1983 = 100

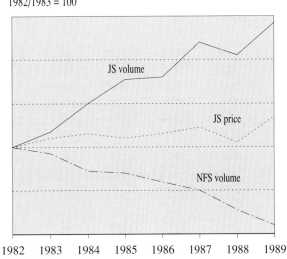

1982   1983   1984   1985   1986   1987   1988   1989

Looking ahead

What of the future? The first thing to be said is that the commercial agencies also live in changing times and have updated their data collection techniques and they are both launching new panels at this point in time. The greatest breakthrough has resulted from the presence of bar codes on virtually all food products. By using these bar codes together with simple hand held terminals, the members of their new panels can identify their purchases much more accurately than ever before. Furthermore, by using telephone communication links, these data can be transmitted quickly and accurately without direct contact with an interviewer. This means that the sample can be spread much more evenly throughout the country minimising the problems that clustered samples may bring to retail measurements.

The next papers give some insight into how the NFS is going to adapt to future needs and also about the problems associated with running the survey. I do not know the extent to which modern technology is being considered but I certainly believe that it could play an important part in improving both the quality and the timeliness of the data.

Secondly I would ask for the results to be published in more meaningful product groupings - or probably sub-groupings so that the integrity of past trends are preserved - so that some of the more interesting and fast changing parts of the diet can be monitored more effectively.

My final plea is for even wider market coverage for example, to include confectionery, soft drinks and snack products and thereby further extend what I have already described as the most broadly based survey of food consumption.

SECTION V

Planned Changes
to the
National Food Survey

CHAPTER 10

Meeting Future Needs

Lesley Yeomans

Introduction

There can be no doubt that the National Food Survey (NFS) has met many of the government's information needs more than adequately for 50 years. But that is not to say that further improvements could not and should not be made. Thus, in 1988, the NFS Committee endorsed a proposal to review certain aspects of the Survey.

Reasons for the Review

There were a number of reasons for a review at this time.

- There have been some dramatic changes in lifestyle in recent years. More women work outside the home; increased ownership of fridges/freezers/microwave ovens; growth of eating out; trend towards 'grazing'; increased demand for convenience/lower calorie/sugar free foods.

- There have been many developments in knowledge and understanding of the relation between diet and health. Undernutrition was a possibility in the past; today the worry is that overconsumption may cause health problems.

These developments raise questions of whether the NFS meets current economic data needs and changing nutritional data needs. Also, whether the NFS methodology is appropriate, efficient, cost-effective and up to date.

- Following the review of the Government Statistical Service in 1980 [1], the cost of the NFS had come under increasing scrutiny.

The fundamental question, therefore, was whether the NFS collects and analyses the right information to meet government's current needs in the most appropriate and cost effective way.

Aims of the Review

The more specific aims of the Review were therefore:

- To ensure that information collected meets the government's current needs.

- To consider whether modifications are required, for example to meet future nutritional uses of the results.

- To ensure that methods and procedures for carrying out the survey are as efficient and up to date as possible.

Scope of the Review

The NFS Committee appointed a steering committee to oversee the review, drawn mainly from the NFS Committee. Working groups were also set up to review three main areas:

- The first group examined uses of the data and, in particular, the relationship between the NFS and Family Expenditure Survey (FES), where there is some overlap in the data collected.

- The nutrition group examined the NFS in terms of monitoring nutritional intakes. They took account of the views of the MAFF Food Safety and Applied Nutrition Consultative Committee and of the health surveys under consideration by the Department of Health.

- The methodology group reviewed the relevance of data collected, size of sample, organisation of fieldwork and coding.

At the outset of the review, the steering committee considered government requirements for data, the extent to which there are gaps and if there were, whether they could be filled by changes to the Survey. The first conclusion we reached was that the NFS does provide the government with economic and nutritional information which is of considerable value for policy purposes.

Current uses of NFS data

(a) **Economic uses**: These are spelled out in more detail earlier but, in relation to national accounts, the NFS results currently provide the basis for aggregating expenditure on household food. This is an important component of the expenditure measure of Gross Domestic Product. Although the basic data for the construction of the retail price index are derived from the Family Expenditure Survey, NFS data are used to provide weights for food subdivisions and the selection of indicator items. NFS data are used by MAFF to provide advice on policy issues such as demand forecasting, implications of EC proposals, market trends and the growth of consumption of new foods, eg. low fat spreads.

(b) **Nutritional uses**: The nutritional uses of NFS data have also been discussed in some detail in other chapters. Nonetheless, it is important to remember that the most important uses are estimates of intake of nutrients, additives, residues and contaminants and the provision of data which illustrate trends over a long period of time.

Gaps in nutritional information

There are, however, two significant gaps in nutritional information provided by the NFS:

- First, the coverage of the Survey is confined to household food and does not provide any information about food bought and eaten outside the home. A number of factors suggest that eating out is an increasingly important part of modern society. The growth of fast food outlets and their success indicates that eating out quickly and conveniently is a major activity. Women work outside the home more, and many people eat out at least once a week. There is more of a social element in eating out as well, and friends and families eat out as a group today rather than visit each other for home prepared food. It is estimated that expenditure on food bought and consumed outside the home has risen from about 20 per cent of expenditure on food ten years ago to around 30 per cent today. If we accept then that food bought and eaten outside the home provides a significant proportion of total food intake, it is clear that the NFS can no longer provide reliable data about total dietary intakes of nutrients, additives etc.

- The second gap in the NFS is that it can say nothing about the nutrient intake or eating behaviour of individuals. All it can do is provide average intakes for all members of a household. In the past it was probably reasonable to assume that all food purchased was eaten by all household members; all meals were eaten together and the same food was eaten by all. Again things are different today; families do not eat together; individuals feed themselves as and when they are at home; individuals within a household may eat special food eg. a vegetarian. It should be made clear, however, that while this is a definite gap, the NFS is not intended to provide data on individuals. Although even here, analysis of NFS data by Professor Chesher is shedding some light on the consumption patterns of different types of individuals within the household.

The Review considered three basic ways in which the NFS could be modified or improved to fill the gaps in the government needs:

- Improve the use of data already collected

- Extend the scope of the NFS

- Improve the survey design

Improve the use of data

(a) **Overlap with the Family Expenditure Survey:** There is some overlap between the NFS and the FES in the collection of information on consumers' expenditure on food. The steering committee examined the question of whether the level of detail in the FES on food expenditure could be reduced, without compromising calculations based on FES data, especially in the context of construction of the Retail Prices Index (RPI). The conclusion was that there seemed to be scope for the level of coding for food in the FES to be reduced.

It was recommended that the reduction in overlap between the NFS and FES should be pursued.

(b) **Data Analysis:** A new database system for the NFS was already being developed when the Review started. It is hoped that the new system will soon be operative. This will represent a significant step forward in that it will allow new food codes to be added which in turn allows greater disaggregation of foods in any analysis. It will also enable easier access to, and analysis of, the NFS data.

It was recommended that full use should be made of the new computer processing system to provide disaggregation of food codes and addtional analyses to meet current economic and nutritional policy needs.

(c) **Commercial sales:** Some sales of data already occur and the committee felt that there is further potential to recoup some of the costs of the survey. However, it was agreed that commercialisation has to be approached with care because of the conflict in objectives between dissemination of information by government and minimising net costs.

It was recommended that the scope for further data sales should be investigated.

Extend the scope of the Survey

As already pointed out, the current scope of the Survey limits the value of the data produced, and may indeed cast doubt on the validity of some of the conclusions drawn. The current limitations relate to;

- soft drinks, confectionery and alcohol

- foods bought and eaten outside the home

The information collected on soft drinks is limited and confectionery and alcoholic drinks are not covered at all. Historically, these items were excluded because they were not generally bought by the housewife and were therefore prone to underestimation. This is no longer seen as a valid objection to their inclusion in the Survey.

It was recommended that confectionery and alcohol should be covered in the NFS and that soft drinks should be integrated into the main analyses.

On the question of food bought and consumed outside the home, extensive investigation has confirmed that there are no sources of comprehensive or reliable data on food purchases away from home. It would be both costly and technically demanding to collect comprehensive data on the *quantity* of all foods bought and consumed outside the home. However, expenditure data together with descriptive details would provide valuable information which would add significantly to the reliability of data on trends in overall eating habits. Collection of such data would increase the costs of the NFS and a feasibility study would be needed to assess the practicality of different methods of collection. The most appropriate method may be to collect information from individuals from a subsample of households participating in the main survey.

It was recommended that information on food bought and eaten away from home should be collected in sufficient detail to fill the present gap in economic and nutritional data.

Improve survey design   The NFS currently achieves a response rate of just under 60 per cent. This is 6 per cent higher than in 1988. The increase is attributed to the sending out of an introductory letter prior to the survey. NFS results are considered statistically valid for main food group analyses. But the sampling error is larger for cells with a small number of observations and results have to be interpreted with some caution. With the introduction of so many new foods there is a need for accurate information from small samples. One way to achieve this would be by increasing the response rate from the current sample. Several means of improving response rates were considered.

(a) **Incentive payments:** These are already used in some government surveys including the FES. However, current response patterns in the NFS indicate that failure to make initial contact with the housewife was a significant factor in not getting a higher response rate. If this is really the problem then incentive payments might have little effect. On the other hand if changes to the Survey require more effort from the housewife, leading to less cooperation, the incentive payments might help to counter any adverse effects on response rate.

(b) **Placement period:** Increasing the period which interviewers have to place the diaries would increase the chance of making contact with the housewife.

(c) **Initial sample:** An alternative to increasing response rates would be to raise the initial sample. But this would however, add substantially to costs.

(d) Extending the record period: This may be another means of collecting data cost effectively. It would also provide additional information on frequency of purchase and would counteract the impact of large purchases at infrequent intervals.

It was recommended that some of these potential methods of improving survey design should be field tested.

Periodicity

At first sight, reducing the frequency of the NFS would save costs, but in practice any savings would be offset by the need to retrain interviewers, coders etc. In addition, reduced frequency would seriously affect the value of the data, given that many uses depend on having reliable up to date information. A continuous NFS allows changes in the average diet to be recognised quickly, thereby enabling the effect of policy changes to be monitored. It was concluded that, on balance, the disadvantages of reducing the frequency of the Survey would outweigh any savings in cost.

It was recommended that the NFS should remain a continuous survey.

Priorities

The steering committee advised that those recommendations which could be most easily introduced and which required minimal additional resources should be implemented as soon as possible. Feasibility studies should be conducted to test the options and determine costs of extending the scope to include food eaten away from home. Feasibility studies should also be conducted to test the options for increasing response and therefore improving the accuracy and reliability of the data.

Progress

MAFF is proceeding to implement the main recommendations as quickly as possible.

- Feasibility studies have been conducted on improving response rates. These indicate that extending the placement period, and evening and weekend placement, would improve the response rate and this change in survey design has now been implemented.

- Feasibility studies are in progress to examine what information could be cost effectively collected on food consumed away from home. It is hoped that these studies will be completed in 1991 and a full scale implementation will begin in 1992.

- As soon as the computer programmes are in place, the NFS will collect data on confectionery and alcohol and integrate the information on soft drinks. This is now expected to be at the beginning of 1992.

REFERENCES

[1] HMSO (1981), Government Statistical Services, Cmnd 8236.

CHAPTER 11

Implementing Change

Robert Redpath

Three organisations are involved in running the National Food Survey (NFS). Overall responsibility for the survey rests with the Ministry of Agriculture, Fisheries and Food (MAFF), which is advised by the National Food Survey Committee. MAFF decides on coverage, undertakes the computer processing and analyses and disseminates the results. The Social Survey Division of the Office of Population Censuses and Surveys (OPCS) is responsible for the design of the survey, the sampling procedures and the testing and implementation of methodological changes. Fieldwork and coding have been contracted out to the private sector, except for one period in the 1950s when this was done by OPCS.

This chapter is concerned with the work of OPCS in the survey operations of sampling, fieldwork and coding. However, in particular, it illustrates the measures that have been taken, and are being taken, to keep the survey up-to-date and to implement the changes recommended by the NFS Committee.

The fieldwork contract

It is considered essential to retender the fieldwork contract periodically to ensure value for money and fair competition. Four organisations have carried out the fieldwork and coding over the 50 years that the survey has been running.

- The London Press Exchange (now Research Services Ltd): 1940-52.

- The Government Social Survey division of the Central Office of Information : 1953-59

- British Market Research Bureau (BMRB) : 1960-90

- Social and Community Planning Research (SCPR) : 1991-

BMRB has had a most distinguished record in carrying out the fieldwork and coding for some 30 years. However, following competitive retendering in 1990, the 1991 contract has been awarded to SCPR and we are confident that the high standards set for the survey will be maintained.

The survey sample

Turning to the survey operations, there is no perfect up to date and complete sampling frame of households in Great Britain. It is necessary, therefore, to settle for population lists which come as close as possible to the ideal. Until 1984, the electoral register was used to select the NFS sample addresses. Since that date, the Small User Postcode Address File (PAF), supplied by the Post Office, has been used as the sample frame. Addresses are selected by computer on the PAF. This saves staff time compared with the former method of manually selecting the sample from electoral registers. Also, the PAF provides better coverage of certain groups not on the register, notably those households with no voters or who have recently moved. The PAF does have disadvantages. Names are not given, only addresses. This means that it is not possible to address advance letters to individuals. Also, it is not possible to distinguish non-private institutions and businesses and this leads to a waste of about 12 per cent of addresses.

In 1985, when the change was made to the PAF, the sample was redesigned so that there were 52 local authorities selected and, within these, 832 postal sectors. Within each of the postal sectors, there were 18 delivery points, which comprise an interviewer's quota of addresses over a 10 day period, giving 14,976 addresses selected each year. A rotating sample design was introduced to provide better estimates of year-to-year changes in sample averages. Each local authority remains in the sample for 24 months and, in each quarter, 6 to 7 local authorities rotate out and are replaced. In 1990, the number of postal sectors was reduced due to cost factors to 780 within 52 local authorities. Although the delivery points sampled was lower, this was largely offset by an improved response rate.

The fieldwork

Unless the interviewers are able to persuade the public to co-operate, there are no survey results to code or analyse. This is an oblique way of stressing the important role that interviewers play in all surveys. Interviewers need to be selected carefully and trained well by their organisations - trained in non-directive techniques, that is to say in learning not to deviate from the question wording and learning how to tactfully probe for missing information. The main measure of an interviewer's performance is the response rate achieved and this depends as much on confidence and morale as on other factors. An important task of those involved in the survey operation is therefore to build up the confidence of interviewers in the survey. In a sense, interviewers are gatekeepers. Before they can convince the public to take part, they need to be convinced themselves of the value of the NFS. For this reason, interviewers are briefed on the main uses of the results, an issue which is covered elsewhere in the proceedings.

However, it is important for interviewers to be aware that the NFS is seen as important by Ministers [1] and to be kept informed of written and oral answers in the House of Commons which refer to the results of the survey as well as articles in newspapers and periodicals.

It helps interviewer confidence and morale if the subject is of interest to the respondent and food prices continue to be a topical subject. One of the nicest compliments that an interviewer can make about a survey is that respondents enjoyed taking part; interviewers frequently hear this about the NFS. Respondents find that they often learn a lot about their shopping by keeping a diary. It is, of course, important that respondents should not change their purchasing patterns during the survey period and interviewers are trained to stress this point. It is also made clear that the survey is voluntary and interviewers are briefed that they should not try to answer political questions which should be referred to their MPs.

One of the main problems which confront interviewers is that they are sometimes suspected of posing as people intending to sell products, or possibly to commit a crime. Interviewers carry identification cards and notify police of the areas in which they are working. It has also been found that sending an advance letter on an OPCS letterhead is helpful and reassuring. Letters are sent first class in official-crested envelopes to avoid possible confusion with junk mail. When the advance letter was first introduced in 1986, response rose from 51 per cent to 58 per cent. This was seen as a more cost-effective means of increasing response than by making payments even though an experiment carried out in 1979 showed that response might be increased by 4-5 per cent if a £2 postal order was offered to those who completed diaries.

Another important element is the leaflet which is given to respondents at the first interview. This includes the pledge of confidentiality which is the absolute base on which the survey operates. This pledge is taken very seriously by interviewers and by all in government. Stringent precautions are taken to ensure that individuals cannot be identified on any data files. Although names and addresses are necessary when the survey is being conducted, these are not entered on the diaries nor on the data tape and are destroyed as soon as is practicable.

The main task of interviewers is to persuade persons to keep a diary for 7 days and to convince them that this is not difficult. An innovation this year is to provide interviewers with a message card in five Asian languages in the event that no-one can speak English at an address. One person in each household is asked to record for seven days the prices, brand names, and weights of all food brought into the home by all members of the household. They are asked to obtain weights of fresh food as bought even if this means weighing it themselves (although sometimes the interviewer helps respondents by weighing food items or indeed by going to a local shop to obtain price or weights). In addition, the menus of up to four main meals, and the whereabouts of all household members when these meals are served, are recorded. Incidentally it is made clear to respondents that they do not have to eat four meals a day, though the diary layout provides for this.

Asking people to keep a diary is one thing, obtaining the necessary detail is another matter. This depends entirely on interviewers being able to probe for the missing detail when they look over the diaries at the checking call and final pick-up call. An entry described as 'milk' is not enough, it is necessary to know if it was skimmed milk, semi-skimmed or whole milk. Similarly, it is necessary to know whether fish is filleted or not and so on. One of the dangers of probing for missing details is that the respondent may feel that she or he is in error or has made mistakes by not providing sufficient detail for the interviewer. The interviewers are briefed to reassure people that participating in the NFS is not an 'A'level exam. Interviewers new to the survey are asked to keep their own household's diaries. This makes it easier for them to introduce the survey to the public.

Nevertheless, the personal checking by interviewers of respondents' diaries is crucial. An experiment carried out in 1979 showed that, if respondents returned their diaries by post without being checked by interviewers, the quality of the data deteriorated. Only one in seven diaries returned by post had complete prices and quantities, compared with one in two diaries where interviewers had personally collected the diaries.

Response rates

The aim in the NFS is to achieve as high response rates as possible not least because of the need to ensure that results are representative of the population. OPCS has on two recent occasions compared the Census characteristics of those who responded to the NFS with those who did not respond. The first was by Kemsley [2] using the 1971 Census data.

A subsequent comparison using 1981 Census data [3] confirmed the earlier results which had shown that there were proportionately more single persons, housewives with full-time employment and married couples without children amongst those households where it had not been possible to make contact (Table 11.1).

Table 11.1
Comparison of 1981
Census characteristics
between households
not contacted and
co-operating households

	Households not contacted %	Co-operating households %
Household size		
Single person	31	16
All other households	69	84
Total	100	100
Number of households	525	2,033
Housewife's employment status		
Full time employee	34	20
Other status	66	80
Total	100	100
Number of households	522	2,029
Family type		
Married, no children	43	31
All other households	57	69
Total	100	100
Number of households	319	1,644

These findings are not surprising; the sub groups who are most likely to slip through the net are those who are less likely to be at home during the day. However, their presence in the survey becomes more and more important as the pattern of eating changes in the direction of convenience foods and meals eaten away from the home. During the first quarter of 1990, an experiment was conducted which allowed interviewers ten days, rather than three, to contact their 18 addresses. The number of days worked was limited to five within the ten day period. This, on average, reduced the non-contact rate from 13 per cent to 8 per cent. The number of co-operating single person households rose, leading to the conclusion that allowing more time to contact the addresses will help to bring into the survey more respondents in the sub-groups which have been under-represented. The change to allow ten days for contact has been introduced for the 1991 Survey.

There is one other group which has difficulty with surveys, and particularly with diary surveys - the elderly. It is common in surveys that response declines the older the respondent after middle age. This is true of the NFS as evidenced from the studies using 1981 Census characteristics (Table 11.2).

Table 11.2
Response to the National
Food Survey by age of
housewife (1981 Census
characteristics)

Age of housewife	Response rate
	%
16-20	67
21-25	61
26-30	64
31-35	62
36-40	64
41-45	58
46-50	57
51-55	56
56-60	53
61-65	44
66-70	45
71 or over	45
Overall average	56
Number of households	3,632

Older people may not wish to co-operate in surveys because they are sick or infirm; they may not feel that the survey is relevant to them. Even if they co-operate they may also worry about doing the diary well. Yet we have evidence that they keep diaries very well. Even with respondents who are not having difficulties, the interviewer returns to make a call half-way through the record-keeping period. It is because of these many calls back to the household that diary surveys are expensive to carry out. In return the interviewer often finds that the elderly person has appreciated the interviewer's company. Interviewers often derive satisfaction from diary surveys because they get to know respondents better than with one-off surveys.

Bringing experienced interviewers together at rebriefings overcomes the isolation they may feel; interviewing is a solitary profession. It enables interviewers to be briefed about new developments in the survey and also for the project officer to be provided with ideas for changes. At the end of the day, however, most agree that it is the interviewer's personality as well as the training which is the key factor in gaining co-operation.

Planned methodological changes

Perhaps the most important methodological change to the NFS for many years is the present brief to add the measurement of all food and drink consumed outside the home to the Survey. One of the obvious changes in the household food consumption in the 1980s has been the increased tendency to eat out as a leisure activity and also the arrival on these shores of the American fast food industry. So eating and drinking outside the home have become an important contributor to nutrient intake.

The major study by OPCS and MAFF on adult nutrition published earlier this year showed that eating out provided 34 per cent of men's and 24 per cent of women's energy value [4]. Therefore this enhancement to the NFS will not be before time. This brief poses quite different methodological needs. Essentially the economists need complete household expenditure information. On the other hand, the food scientists and nutritionists are ideally interested in actual consumption of food and drink by individuals not households. Additionally, they are interested in considerably greater detail about what is eaten and how much is eaten.

These two sets of requirements are partly compatible but not entirely so. Experiments have been started in which everyone aged 11 and over in a household has been asked to keep a week's diary of all food and drink consumed outside the home. Additionally, the main record-keeper has kept records of the expenditure by, and on behalf of, children under the age of 11. Surprisingly, in the first stage experiment, the response to the Survey went up rather than down as a result of these additional tasks. Further tests on a far larger sample are needed to be certain about the effect on response but the results so far have been encouraging. Basically households see the sense of recording the food and drink they consume outside the home as well as inside the home. And this in turn gives the interviewers confidence that it can work.

Another enhancement will take place when respondents are asked to record alcoholic drink and confectionery brought home. Estimates of expenditure on alcoholic drink and confectionery based on the Family Expenditure Survey (FES) are consistently understated.

One of the reasons why expenditure on confectionery is understated is that diary record-keeping on the FES is restricted to those aged 16 and over. By asking children aged 11 and over to keep diaries, this deficiency may be largely overcome. However, this assumes that the child believes that the diary will not be seen by a parent; it is made clear that diaries are confidential to each person, adults included. It is amazing how food bought and consumed can be a sensitive subject within families.

The same concerns, of course, surround the recording of alcohol consumption which is estimated to be consistently under-recorded in the FES when compared with national accounts figures based on Customs and Excise data. A considerable amount of research was carried out into the possible reasons for the discrepancy between the FES measurement of alcohol consumption and the national accounts and concluded that the main reason was that very heavy drinkers did not participate in the survey.

Inevitably, it is easier to obtain the expenditure data on eating and drinking out than to try to measure the actual consumption of individuals which is needed for food scientists and nutritionists. The NFS can not be expected to serve as a full-fledged nutrition survey, such as that proposed in the programme of National Dietary Surveys of Individuals referred to in the first paper. However, data collected for the NFS can be used to update the nutritional data collected in these benchmark surveys.

The continuing methodological problem is how to measure portion sizes of food and drink consumed outside the home. A visit last summer to the United States Department of Agriculture indicated that there is no easy answer to this problem as members of the public are likely to find that very precise measurement, ie: by polaroid cameras, measuring spoons, rulers, etc, is likely to be intrusive and either affect response or change behaviour. For this reason, the initial enhancement will focus on the considerable amount of detailed breakdown of types of food and drink for nutritional analysis, as well as the easier measures of quantity, eg, numbers of rashers of bacon, sausages, eggs, chops, etc.

As always with any major methodological change such as this, it takes time to build up interviewer confidence that such data can be collected. Miracles do not happen instantaneously, if at all, and pragmistism is the name of the game with all voluntary diary surveys. So it is expected that the data will improve incrementally over time and that there will be problems along the way.

Coding

Very little has been said about coding. It is an important and specialised area. Coders, through their experience, become adept at sensing mis-recorded weights of packaged and tinned goods. Even after the careful checking by interviewers there are gaps in the data which necessitate either re-contacting the record-keeper or else imputing. The NFS sets very high standards of acceptable recording. For example a diary can be rejected if there is not a breakdown of individual items and individual prices and weights are not given separately. An example would be £2.50 spent on fruit and vegetables. Here, the detail is not sufficient for analysis. Coders have to complete coding within 20 working days from the end of the fieldwork period. This, as with the short contact period interviewers have, indicates the pressure to produce timely results not only for national accounts and the Retail Price Index (RPI) but also for press releases and policy analysis. In terms of other major government surveys , the NFS data must be amongst the quickest to release results.

In closing, it is relevant to recall an account of the methodology of another diary survey.

" The method of inquiry was as follows. Notebooks were prepared and given to the families whose diet it was wished to study. On the first page of these the housewife was asked to write down the total income received during the week from all sources, in money or in kind (including gifts), the age and sex of all members of the household and the sum paid for rent. There were fourteen pages, two for each day of the week. On one of these pages the housewife was asked to keep an account of all money spent, showing the kind and quantity of goods purchased each day and the prices paid. On the opposite page she was asked to state what the family had to eat and drink at each meal and the number of persons present."

That methodology sounds very familiar and could be the NFS. In fact it was fromRowntree's classic study carried out in York in 1899 [6]. Table 11.3 gives examples of the entries of expenditure on food, as well as a page of menus served to a family of seven (father, mother and five children) during a week ending 30 June 1899.

Table 11.3
Diary extract from
Rowntree's study of
household food
purchases

		Purchases during week ending 30 June 1899
Friday	1½ st flour	1s 10 d.
	¼ st wheatmeal	4d.
	yeast	1d.
	1 lb butter	10d.
	2½ lbs bacon	1s.
	6 oz tea	6d.
	1 lb currants	3d.
	1 lb lard	4d.
	1 ¼ lbs fish	4d.
	1 tin condensed milk	5½d.
Saturday	4 lbs beef	1s 7 ½d.
	5 lbs sugar	9d.
	8 eggs	6d.
	baking powder	1d.
	lemons	2d.
Sunday	milk	1d.
Tuesday	yeast	1d.
Thursday	lettuce	1d.

Table 11.3 continued

	Menu of meals provided during week ending 30 June 1899		
	Breakfast	Dinner	Tea
Friday	Brown and white bread, butter, tea	Fish, bread, tea	Bread,butter, onions, tea
Saturday	Bacon, bread, tea	Eggs, bread, butter, tea	Bread, dripping, onions, tea
Sunday	Bacon, bread, tea	Potato pie, potatoes, cabbage	Bread, butter, currant cake, tea
Monday	Porridge, bread, butter, tea	Potato pie	Bread, butter, currant cake, tea
Tuesday	Brown and white bread, butter, tea	Meat, bread, tea	Bread, butter, dripping, tea
Wednesday	Brown and white bread, butter, tea	Bread, bacon, tea	Bread, butter, dripping, tea
Thursday	Porridge, bread, butter, tea	Bacon, bread, bread pudding, tea	Bread, butter, lettuce, tea

The methodology of diary surveys has not changed much since Rowntree, even if the diets we now enjoy have changed a great deal. Diary surveys still are, and will continue to remain, a simple but powerful tool for monitoring how we all live.

REFERENCES

[1] Market Research Society (Winter 1990), *The Survey Interview*, Market Research Journal, pp 33-35.

[2] Kemsley, W F F (November 1976), *National Food Survey - a Study of Differential Reponse Based on a Comparison of the 1971 Census*, Statistical News 35, pp 18-22.

[3] Redpath, R U and Elliot, D (February 1988), *National Food Survey - a Second Study of Differential Response comparing Census characteristics of NFS respondents and non-respondents; also a comparison of NFS and FES response bias*, Statistical News 80, pp 6-10.

[4] Gregory, J, Foster, K, Tyler, H and Wiseman, M (1990), *The Dietary and Nutritional Survey of British Adults*, HMSO.

[5] Kemsley, W F F and Redpath, R U (1980), *Family Expenditure Survey Handbook*, HMSO.

[6] Rowntree, B (1902), *Poverty - a Study of Town Life*, Seebohm MacMillan.

Structure of the
National Food Survey

Introduction

The National Food Survey is a continuous sampling enquiry into the domestic food consumption and expenditure of private households in Great Britain. Each household which participates does so voluntarily, and without payment, for one week only. By regularly changing the households surveyed, information is obtained continuously throughout the year apart from a short break at Christmas.

Information provided by households

The sole informant in each household is the person, female or male, principally responsible for domestic arrangements. For convenience, that person is referred to as the 'housewife'. She (or he) keeps a 7-day diary, with guidance from an interviewer, of all the food entering the home each day that is intended for human consumption; the Survey therefore currently excludes meals out and pet food. The following details are noted for each item; the description, the quantity (in either imperial or metric units) and - in respect of purchases - the cost. Food obtained free from a farm or other business owned by a household member or from a garden on allotment is recorded only at the time it is used. To avoid the double counting of purchases, gifts of food are excluded if they were bought by the donating households. Also currently excluded from the Survey are a few items which individual family members often buy for themselves without coming to the attention of the housewife - the Survey's sole informant; these are chocolates, sugar confectionery, and soft and alcoholic drinks.[1]

---

1   Since 1975, particulars have been obtained of soft dinks bought for the household supply. The results are presented in the annual report but the information is excluded from the main analyses because of the likelihood of bias from under-recorrding.

As well as the detail about the foods entering the household, the housewife also notes which persons (including visitors) are present at each meal together with a description of the type (but not the quantities) of food served. This enables an approximate check to be made between the foods served and those acquired during the week. Records are also kept of the number and nature (whether lunch, dinner, etc) of the meals obtained outside the home by each member of the household; this is used in the nutritional calculations. No information is currently collected, however, about the cost or composition of meals taken outside the home although, exceptionally, the quantity of school milk consumed by children is recorded.

Finally, on a separate questionnaire, details are entered of the characteristics of the family and its members but names are not collected. The identities of addresses are strictly confidential. They are known only to those who are involved with selecting the sample and carrying out the fieldwork. They are not even divulged to the Ministry of Agriculture, Fisheries and Food which is responsible for analysing and reporting the Survey results.

As the Survey records only the quantities of food entering the household and not the amount actually consumed, it cannot provide meaningful frequency distributions of households classified according to levels of food eaten or of nutrition. However, averaged over sufficient households, the quantities recorded should equate with consumption (in the widest possible sense, including waste food discarded or fed to pets) provided purchasing habits are not upset and there is no general accumulation or depletion of household food stocks.

The National Food Survey is selected to be representative of mainland Great Britain (including the Isle of Wight but not the Scilly Isles nor the islands of Scotland). In recent years a three-stage stratified random sample scheme has been used, the first stage of which involves the selection of local authority districts as the primary sampling units (PSUs). An eighth of the local authority districts are retired and replaced each quarter (reselection being possible) and once selected, remain in the Survey for eight consecutive quarters before being retired. The number of local authority districts included in the Survey for sampling purposes is 52 at any one time. The second stage of selection procedure involves the selection of postal sectors within each of the districts and the third stage the selection of 18 delivery points from each postal sector. The delivery points are drawn from the Small Users Postcode Address File (PAF) using interval sampling from a random origin.

The 52 local authority districts selected are randomly divided into two sets of 26. The two sets are worked in alternate 21 day intervals with two postal sectors covered during each 21 day interval. Thus, in the first interval, 52 postal sectors from one set of 26 local authority districts are worked and in the second 21 day interval 52 postal sectors from the other set are worked. Each set of local authority districts is worked for eight 21 day intervals throughout the year, therefore the sample covers 336 days out of the 365 days in the year.

Nutritional analysis of survey results

The energy value and nutrient content of food obtained for consumption in the home are evaluated using special tables for food composition. The nutrient conversion factors were originally based on values given in *The Composition of Foods* [1] but are thoroughly revised each year for two reasons. First, to reflect changes in nutrient values resulting from new methods of food production, handling and fortification. Second, to reflect changes in the structure of the food categories used in the Survey - for example changes in the relative importance of the many products grouped under 'breakfast cereals'.

The nutrient factors used make allowance for inedible materials such as the bones in meat and the outer leaves and skins of vegetables; for certain foods, such as potatoes and carrots, allowance is also made for seasonal variations in this wastage and/or nutrient content. Further allowance is made for the expected cooking losses of thiamin and vitamin C; average thiamin retention factors are applied to appropriate items within each major food group and the (weighted) average loss over the whole diet is estimated to be about 20 per cent; the losses of vitamin C are set at 75 per cent for green vegetables and 50 per cent for other vegetables. However, no allowance is made for the wastage of edible food. The exception is when the adequacy of the diet is being assessed in comparison with the recommended intakes. Then, the assumption is made that in each type of household, 10 per cent of all foods - and hence of all nutrients available for consumption - is either lost through wastage or spoilage in the kitchen or on the plate, or fed to domestic pets.[2]

The energy content of the food is calculated from the protein, fat and available carbohydrate (expressed as monosaccharide) contents using the respective conversion factors, 4, 9 and 3.75 kcal per gram. It is expressed both in kilocalories and megajoules (1,000 kcal = 4.184 MJ). Niacin is expressed both as free niacin and as niacin equivalent; the latter value includes one-sixtieth of the tryptophan content of the protein in the food. Vitamin A activity is expressed as micrograms of retinol equivalent, that is the sum of the weights of retinol and one-sixth of the β-carotene. Fatty acids are grouped according to the number of double bonds present, that is into saturated, monosaturated and poly-unsaturated fatty acids. For the diet as a whole, the total fatty acids

---

2 An enquiry into the amounts of potentially edible food which are thrown away or fed to pets in Great Britain recorded an average wastage of about 6 per cent of households' food supplies [2]. However, this is considered likely to be a minimum estimate, and the convential Survey deduction of 10 per cent has been retained thereby preserving continuity with earlier years.

constitute about 95 per cent of the weight of the fat. This proportion varies slightly for individual foods, being lower for dairy fats with their greater content of short-chain acids and a little higher for most other foods.

REFERENCES

[1] Paul, A A and Southgate, D A T (1978), *McCance and Widdowson's The Composition of Foods*, 4th edition, Ministry of Agriculture, Fisheries and Food and Medical Research Council, HMSO.

[2] Wenlock, R W, Buss, D H, Derry, B J and Dixon, E J (1980), *Household Food Wastage in Britain*, British Journal of Nutrition, 43, pp 53-70.